One Little Finger

To dear Geeta aunty,
Thanks for all your support.
Happy Reading...
Love,
Malini

Malini Chib

SAGE www.sagepublications.com
Los Angeles • London • New Delhi • Singapore • Washington DC

First published in 2011 by

SAGE Publications India Pvt Ltd
B1/I-1 Mohan Cooperative Industrial Area
Mathura Road, New Delhi 110 044, India
www.sagepub.in

SAGE Publications Inc
2455 Teller Road
Thousand Oaks, California 91320, USA

SAGE Publications Ltd
1 Oliver's Yard, 55 City Road
London EC1Y 1SP, United Kingdom

SAGE Publications Asia-Pacific Pte Ltd
33 Pekin Street
#02-01 Far East Square
Singapore 048763

Published by Vivek Mehra for SAGE Publications India Pvt Ltd, typeset in 12/16 pt Adobe Garamond by Diligent Typesetter, Delhi and printed at Chaman Enterprises, New Delhi.

Library of Congress Cataloging-in-Publication Data Available

ISBN: 978-81-321-0632-6 (PB)

The SAGE Team: Rekha Natarajan, Swati Sengupta, Sanjeev Kumar Sharma and Deepti Saxena

Cover photograph by Avinash Gowarikar.

This book is dedicated to my mother.

Mother,
Thank you
For constantly pushing me all my life,
For always being there for me,
For making your life centric to me.
Thank you for sharing and giving me so much,
Motivating me and giving me a full life.

This book would have not been possible without your support.

In Memory of

My nephew Ishan Bose-Pyne, who left us at the age of 16 through an accident in Los Angeles, while I was finishing my last chapter. He loved sitting on my wheelchair and whizzing around Regents' Park and feeding the squirrels with me, not at all fazed out or scared of falling. I loved carrying him like that, it was my first experience of being a mother and holding a child, he will always remain with me.

Contents

Reflections

Acknowledgements

Although I managed to finish this book, it was a long arduous effort, and there is a tale to tell. It needed quite a bit of editing from several people. The book would not have been possible without the support and help of my mother, Mithu Alur. At the same time, the finalization of endless proof-reading and corrections was possible because of the indefatigable work it received from my friend, Theresa D'Costa, and Lucas Baretto's secretarial help.

I would like to acknowledge and thank the SAGE team for making this book happen—Sugata Ghosh for believing in this project, my deep thanks and appreciation to Rekha Natarajan for her skilled editing. It was a great experience working with them. Thank you for all your assistance.

One

ROOTS

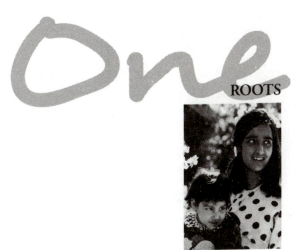

Proving the Doctors Wrong

The month was July, the year 1966. The place—Woodlands Nursing Home, Calcutta. Looking back, I realize that at the time of my birth, knowledge about disability was rare. I was told that my mother was in labour for a lengthy 40-hour period. During the process, the umbilical chord got stuck around my neck, resulting in a lack of oxygen to my brain and a few seconds of that (known by the medical term of *anoxia*) eventuated in giving me a lifetime of a severe disabling condition (condition not disease!) called Cerebral Palsy. The birth was hugely traumatic, and the pediatrician in charge kept repeating to himself *'it was a mistake I should have carried out a caesarean...lets see if she survives...I am not sure if she will survive...at the most 72 hours'*.

I survived. Apparently, I was a beautiful baby. I had very fair complexion with large eyes and black hair. I went home from the hospital to my grandparents' house, where I had a full-time Australian nurse who called me 'Rosebud' and 'Princess'. There was a beautiful nursery which awaited me, filled with lovely bright toys that I could look at and play with.

But I did not play. My mother's writings describe me as being weak and not doing much. The little effort necessary for sucking the bottle was enough to tire me and I slept all day. I got terrified by noises. For weeks and months, I was cooed at and admired by my family. *I remained passive.*

My mother began to worry. Why did everything make me so scared? I was startled easily and cried a lot. The doctors said it was a result of the birth trauma I had experienced. A year-and-a-half went by. I grew older and was not keeping up with the milestones. Everyone began to wonder whether there was something wrong with me. Why did I not move much? Why did I not sit up, or roll over, or kick my legs like other babies?

My parents were very young and went berserk with worry and anxiety. They were supported by a loving, caring family who wanted to do everything for me. They moved from one doctor to the other and saw over a dozen specialists for a correct diagnosis. My mother clung to the hope that everything would be alright. She often argued with my father and wondered why her beautiful baby was considered not normal.

During this time in India, my mother went through a period of depression. The concept of a handicap was new to her and her family. She was confused and did not know what to expect. She almost believed the doctors who thought I was mentally handicapped.

There were endless examinations done by doctors. I am told that I hated these examinations. The doctors pulled at my limbs and I shrieked with fright. But my mother writes that they remained cold, silent, strange, and unsmiling in their white coats; not talking or chatting with me or my parents. I clung to my mother crying hopelessly. I must have thought I was being punished.

From these visits, it was learnt that there was some matter with me. A diagnosis emerged at last when I was five months old and my parents were told quite brusquely that I was a spastic and had Cerebral Palsy. My poor mother began to cry. She had no idea what that meant or what the implications were. My father was busy consoling her. Soon they began to read up on the condition and question the people close to them about it. They found out that the motor cells of my brain were damaged and I suffered from a lack of co-ordination and balance. During birth, I got suffocated while trying to come out of my mother's womb and the lack of oxygen had damaged my brain. I was going to face difficulty in performing tasks that needed physical skills. Therefore, activities like walking, talking and even eating and swallowing were going to be enormous efforts for me.

Every doctor my parents met in India told them that I would be a vegetable and nothing could be done for me. The doctors confidently told them that the damage to my brain was irreversible.

My parents refused to believe them. They did not give up on believing in me. My mother was taught exercises to carry out with me. I began my exercises from the age of seven months. I was taught how to stretch my hand out and reach for a toy, as I was unable to even do that. I was taught how to balance myself when carried, how to roll over and generally, all the milestones that a normal child does easily and automatically. These exercises became a daily pattern of my life, like breathing in and breathing out, eating and sleeping. The exercises had to be done and my parents and family spent a great deal of time on me. My parents did not give up. They were fighters. Besides being fighters, they were focused and very conscientious about the routines.

I am told that I revolted quite often. Maybe, I questioned my dreary life and why I could not run, play and explore my surroundings. I was pushed, wheedled, persuaded and coerced by my mother. Lots of bribes were used and I often got a chocolate bar if I did well.

The great thing is that although I could not do very much with my body, I understood all that happened around me. I even followed the stories my parents read to me. My father said I remembered each story so well that if he tried to skip a couple of pages to end the story quicker, I would *know* and start agitating and pointing to the book until he went back to the story. I could follow everything that people said to me though I could not respond.

Some people could not understand that although I did not speak, I could comprehend. These people had nothing to say to me. The children too could not understand why I did not play the usual games with them. They too left me alone. Mother recalls at one birthday party, I was depressed a great deal as everybody left me alone. The hostess gave all the kids their going away presents of balloons, hats and whistles while leaving me out. She said she was sorry but she did not think I would be able to play with them properly. I think the worst thing that can happen to a child with a disability is to leave them alone and not even talk to them.

When I went out, I became conscious of all the stares that I provoked, the hushed whisperings when I appeared, the unsolicited advice that was proffered. My mother writes that when I met strangers, or entered a room full of people, I began to put my head down, terribly conscious of myself and the fact that I was different from others. The thought that somebody may notice I was present and ask something about me, was mortifying.

However, I was fortunate I came from a privileged and well educated family. Both my grandfather had been educated in England, and my great aunt was Lotika Sarkar—the first woman from India to have gone to Newnham College, Cambridge. My father and my uncle had both had their higher education at Cambridge as well.

My uncle, Samiran, was working as a Physician at the Royal Post-Graduate Medical School at Hammersmith Hospital, London. He consulted leading pediatricians, Dr Jack Tizard of Great Ormond Street Hospital, London; Dr Douglas Gairdner of Addenbrooks Hospital, Cambridge and Dr Philip Evans. He told them that the Indian doctors did not know much and were extremely negative about my condition which they had diagnosed as spastic with mental retardation. Considering it was brain damage, they had concluded nothing could be done, even in England.

The doctors looked through the papers and were most compassionate and encouraging. Dr Gairdner suggested that I should go to a special school called Roger in Ascham, Cambridge. My father was convinced about England. He knew that in the areas of medicine and education, England was far superior to India. My parents decided to wind up their life in India and take me to England for my treatment.

It was a momentous decision for them in many ways. My parents had to give up their large house. My father resigned from his job at Tata at a crucial moment, as he was just beginning to do well. Tatas played a pivotal role and gave my parents all help.

Every piece of furniture that had been personally designed by my mother had to go—the car, crockery, cutlery—as the entire household was wound up. My parents gave up their cushy life and said goodbye to their friends and their life as they had known it.

Mother went ahead with me to England. We stayed with the Nundys in their delightful little house in Cambridge, called Springfield which belonged to Bishop Montefiore. It was a two bedroom semi-detached house with a front and back garden, where Samiran and Ranjit would later spend long summer evenings making plans about the future. My father was extremely concerned about my development. I remember watching important events on TV like the landing on the moon, sitting together with my parents, uncles and aunt. We were a happy joint family. My aunt, Mita, was a year younger than mother and had not felt the need of getting a degree after she left school. However, on reaching Cambridge, she began to study again, registering for the 'A' level programme. Two other aunts of mine, Brinda and Radhika, were in London. Radhika took up a course in speech pathology and communication.

I was apparently happy at the school I went to. From my special school in Cambridge called Roger Ascham School, I moved to a school at Cheyne Walk, Chelsea in London. Cheyne was the best special school for children from infant level to seven years. I had a fairly complex IQ test given to me by a well-known psychologist, Agatha Bowley. One of the complicated tasks involved a pole with six balls. I was shown what to do. Each ball was put into the hollow pole. Then at the other end, the pole was lifted and the balls would come out. Three or four balls were repeatedly put into the pole and the pole was pulled upwards to show the ball coming out of the other end. I was then asked to do this. Apparently, without too much ado, I believe I took each ball and began putting it into the pole. I put in one slowly, then the next one very slowly, then the next without lifting the pole up.

Meanwhile, my parents, who were watching, were full of trepidation thinking I had not understood the task at all. Finally, with meticulous care I put in all six balls, and then lifted the pole up only once as all the little balls came tumbling out. I figured why bother with the pole each time, but do the whole task in one go. Amidst applause I continued with other such tasks. In the report which resulted from the IQ test, I was judged to be above average, showing initiative and imagination. My IQ was 120. I did have irreversible brain damage but I was not mentally handicapped. In fact, I was normal and above average in intelligence. A graphic description commonly used to describe children like me in England was apparently 'an intelligent mind with a disobedient body'. My parents were full of pride and that night the family opened a bottle of champagne. Clearly, the doctors in India were wrong to have said that I would be a vegetable.

At Cheyne, I received the best treatment and educational management. My physiotherapist was a person called Noreen Hare who was very fond of me yet quite firm with me. In the early days, I hated having to go to her and would try my tricks; I resisted her stubbornly. I would bawl loudly and people would run to see if I was hurt. It was quite a battle between Noreen and me, as I refused to be touched and pulled. Fortunately, Noreen won the battle. It was a great deal of work learning to walk, learning to speak and training my spastic muscles to move. When Noreen was not working with me, I explored and examined all the toys on my own in the classroom. Apparently,

I was a bit of a loner. All the while I counted the hours when my mum would come and fetch me home.

I progressed immensely at Cheyne. I sat up, began to crawl, pulled myself upto furniture and could walk when aided. The approach to me was different. It was a kind, encouraging and understanding team of professionals who dealt with me.

Educationally too, I prospered. In the evenings I played memory games and master mind with my father. I had a very good memory and my father told me that I beat him most of the time. He used to love recounting this story to all his friends.

I received excellent stimulation and exposure both at home and at school. I travelled with my parents all around Britain and Europe. My mother, being very delicate, could not stand the English winter, so we went to the Bahamas, where my paternal grandparents lived, for the winter vacations. My grandfather was Director of Tourism there. They lived in style with a swimming pool on the grounds of the house. The people my mother met with were wealthy Americans, average age 50–60, and retired, who only talked of their wealth. Once a lady came with her white Pomeranian dog that wore a diamond collar; the dog sat on a high chair, joining us at the table. I was also on a high chair. Every meal was a nine-course affair. Being a very eager two-year old, I had to taste each and every course sitting on a high chair next to my parents. I also swam a great deal with my father. I felt grand, confident and ready to conquer the world.

My school at Cheyne Walk overlooked the tranquil expanse of greenery of Battersea Park and the River Thames. Battersea Park is very well located in south London. The park has a fascinating history and has some major landmarks nearby, such as Battersea Power Station and the Battersea Dog's Home. Surrounding the school were Edwardian houses which had individually manicured patches of greenery and when the flowers were in full bloom, the gardens look ravishing. A statue of one of England's finest statesmen who in his lifetime gained a reputation as a leading Renaissance humanist scholar, Sir Thomas Moore, was positioned right in front of the school.

The school offered a variety of activities that included Physiotherapy, Speech and Occupational therapy, along with education, all under one roof. Education was fun. As toddlers, we were always playing and experimenting with water sand and clay. One of my oldest memories of my school were that we were taken to an adventure playground situated round the corner, every Thursday. I loved being taken up to tree houses, going into tunnels and coming out and climbing what looked like huge jungle gyms.

The new approach treated parents differently than they did in India. With the nurturing, kindness and support I got at Cheyne in England, I grew from strength to strength.

My mother too developed. She stopped weeping. In the early days, my father said she would frequently cry, but she became stronger as she saw me improve and be handled so effectively with a new approach. My father then helped to persuade her to become a professional. He filled in her enrolment forms to read for a postgraduate diploma course at the Institute of Education, University of London, so that she could become a special educationist. She did well. She later became one of the first and finest special educationists in India.

Cheyne was a Teaching Hospital. Doctors, paramedicals and other connected professionals were constantly in the lecture halls going through courses about their approach and the management of Cerebral Palsy. Apparently, I was loved by all the doctors during the demonstrations. I was frequently the guinea pig because I was a good little guinea pig and performed very well before the crowd. I am told that after the demonstrations, I would blow kisses to the audience amidst applause.

Meanwhile, I was constantly being groomed. I was taught how to read at the age of two by my mother and aunt through a flash card method; they made cards for all the common words and taught them to me. I had all the attention I needed when I was young from the family. My father at that time worked at Gallop Poll in Regent's Street. After work, he would go to the well-known toyshop in Carnaby Street called Galt and buy complicated games like the Memory Game and Master Mind. After learning one or two techniques on how to win, I regularly beat my father and uncle. My uncle would carry me around on his shoulder and point out everything to me. Another aunt of mine became a professional speech therapist from the Hampstead School and she would tell us about communication. They all treated me normally and spent quality time speaking to me about life and reading me stories. I could not have had a more cognitively stimulating environment. These early years shaped me and I did very well in school.

Emotionally too, those were happy, sunny days, full of fun and laughter. My parents had plenty of *joie de vivre*. I, too, was a very happy baby, except when I parted from them. The three of us prospered and blossomed.

At 29, my father became the youngest Director of Gallup Poll and the only Indian to be one. My mother became a professional special education teacher and began work with mentally handicapped adults at an institute in Balham (south London). This training gave her a lot more information about my condition. Knowing more about it, she was more emotionally settled. My father's decision to move to England was proved right. As for me, I enjoyed my home, school, my birthdays and holidays. I bloomed and laughed.

After living in Cromwell Road for over a-year-and-half, my father brought a three-bedroom house with a large back garden in Ham, a suburb of Richmond. Our home was No. 58, Broughten Avenue in Ham. Ham is a beautiful place—full of quiet lanes with plenty greenery. The front garden had a weeping willow tree. My mother's song of choice when she saw this tree was 'there is a tavern in the town'. My mother was now her usual cheerful bundle of energy and loved singing to me.

Richmond Park was our favourite haunt, where we would often have picnics while watching the deer. The area was quiet and one could hear the birds sing. Another familiar sound was the ice cream man's van. I used to wait the whole afternoon for him as I loved to gorge on Italian ice cream. The population of the village we lived in was small. Everyone knew me and would come up and chat. My uncle and aunt had also bought a house earlier in Kingfisher Drive which was only a 100 yards from us. I could run to them using my outdoor walker which Cheyne had provided. Life in Ham was fun for the Nundys and the Chibs. Every Sunday, Samiran and Ranjit would normally have a glass of beer at the local pub, while waiting for their clothes to be washed at the launderette.

My parents were keen to have a second child but they were also worried that something would go wrong, so they consulted Professor Brown. He advised them that it would be better if mother had a type of caesarian known as an elective caesarian, where the surgery was scheduled to be performed at an appointed date decided beforehand.

My little brother was born into this pleasant and salubrious atmosphere. Psychologists, social workers and rehabilitators of disabled people and families, always advise parents with a disabled first-born in order to have a second child. They believe that another child can help to stabilize the family. When a couple's first child is disabled, they are always afraid to have a second child and often end up not having another. This to me is a shame because a second child brings normality to everyone's lives as my brother did to ours.

Mother proudly delivered a boy on the 20th July. He weighed 7 lbs and was beautiful to look at. Fair complexioned, dark eyed, well shaped lips and jet black hair. The whole neighbourhood came to know about it as our next door neighbour, Bernice, who was very close to us, ran around screaming with delight and joy.

I went to see him in my best party dress with a present, which I thought I must take. I bought a lovely red toy car for my day old brother. I loved my brother dearly. He had a wonderful temperament. My mother said he would always wait patiently for his early morning milk until after I left for school.

He was very sunny-natured and would happily stay with my grandmother, aunt, or uncle if my parents went out. I did not feel any tinge of jealousy when my parents were with Nicky. I only felt joy. He was named Nikhilesh and we called him Nikhil affectionately. My parents proudly chose this name. Nikhil was normal. He was going to play a very special part in our lives.

I continued to attend Cheyne Walk. Cheyne had given me a solid foundation and educationally, I was above normal. Although I went to a special school, my parents always saw to it that I did what any other child of that age would do. I was read to, constantly. My father would often call me a genius after losing a master mind game, and together we tried out tougher games.

Life, however, became difficult for my parents. To manage two kids took up all their time and they hardly had any time for each other. They had both been through a great deal of stress and it was beginning to show. After Nikhil was born, my parents decided to return to India. Physically, they could not cope with two children. Domestic work was hard work for both my parents, especially, for my mother. Also, after six years of staying in England, they yearned for their own country. They felt that they needed to contribute to India as they were both hugely nationalistic.

They missed India and decided to go back.

This was a difficult goodbye for me. London was the place where I had blossomed, where I acquired stability with excellent management for the first time since my birth. I had learnt to read, do well intellectually and had begun to walk. People here loved and accepted me for what I was.

My parents and I did not realize then that a dark period in our lives was approaching, and there were momentous challenges that awaited us in India.

Birth of a Movement

We returned home to Bombay from England filled with thoughts of how wonderful getting back home was going to be, but we were in for a rude shock. Seven years ago, the doctors had said that I would be a vegetable and the situation of ignorance still continued. There were no schools for me. They were still very ignorant about their approach to people with disabilities.

To begin with, I went to a leading Children's Hospital for my treatment. They spoke about me in front of me, often not directly addressing me. They poked and examined me as if I did not feel any pain. Well, I was just a patient and not a human being.

'Does she need a collar to hold her head up?'

'I think homeopathy will help her ... why don't you try that?'

'Oh, she cannot hold a pencil, she cannot tie her shoe laces, she cannot undress or dress independently and cannot feed herself.'

The paramedical staff treated me as if I did not have ears or could not understand. To them, I was a non-thinking person who needed fixing and fitting into the mould of being normal.

I hated the whole experience.

My experiences in Cheyne, of their kindness and sensitivity towards me were fresh in my mind. I well remember that the Cheyne staff had been so nurturing, friendly, warm, sensitive and egalitarian. They had treated me as a child first, not a handicapped child. I did not have the words to express my deep grief and sadness; nobody thought I could understand. Being only six, I collapsed into tears; of course I could understand everything they said. I would wonder why they were so negative about me. The more I thought of it, the worse I felt. These people were different. These people were rough, hierarchical, domineering, intimidating and wanted to prove that they were superior professionals. Their treatment of me made me weep. My mother and grandmother wept with me. What were we to do?

My distress and the trauma of being with people so completely different affected my mother terribly. She had no one to talk to about her grief and became quite distraught. The social attitude towards me affected her badly, and she became isolated with her grief and suffering. She became introspective with the situation. She started questioning what was happening to other children with multiple disabilities.

It was then that the idea of setting up a model of a school based on what she had experienced in England dawned on her. A replica school like the one I went to at Cheyne Walk, which she would develop within the Indian context and to suit Indian needs.

It was the era of special education in England when I was a child. All over the world, disability was steeped in the medical model of curing persons with disabilities. This is what my mother had been exposed to. It was at that historical period in the early 1970s that the first school called The Centre for Special Education was set up in Bombay. My mother, who came from a culturally rich background, put in her valuable contributions to the model. For social and emotional development, I remember we had plays, sports, painting and art and crafts. Greeting cards were printed in the early days and Frank Simoes, a well-known person from the advertising world, developed this with her. Exhibitions called 'I Can' were held to show the artistic skill of children with disability.

The centre was opened on Gandhiji's birthday, 2 October 1972, in a very beautiful bungalow on army territory, in an idyllic setting overlooking the Arabian Sea. The then Prime Minister, Mrs Indira Gandhi had helped in getting this building.

My father, in fact, the whole family reacted in a very positive manner and came forward to support the initiative. They all set about working for establishing services for the school, with my mother taking the lead. Mother was a special educationist but for the treatment, she needed a qualified therapist who had worked with Cerebral Palsy before. That is when Pam Stretch came in. Mother had approached VSO (Voluntary Services Overseas), United Kingdom (UK). Months later, a letter arrived from a Pam Stretch. Pam was looking for a posting in Africa or India. When she received the letter from VSO about our needs, Pam excitedly accepted our job in India and we were lucky to have Pam. Her training had been in London. Coincidently, she had spent a six weeks' training period in Cheyne Walk while I was there but our paths had never crossed.

Pam had several years of experience in the service of children with Cerebral Palsy and was a much needed input at my mother's special school. On 24 September 1974, Pam arrived by British Airways. Pam was round, comely and warm. She had an infectious laugh and saw life in a humorous way. She was hugely sincere, very kind and generous and had a real knack in serving humanity. Pioneering work is a round the clock job and Pam and mother needed to spend more time together. Pam moved in with us and helped to bring us up. For her, we became her Indian nuclear family. Pam initially was to stay for two years but instead, stayed on for 22 years.

Pam and mother bonded extremely well as they were both quite alike. Their desire to serve, to reach out to others so willingly and with such ease, to accept without questioning, brought in crowds of parents and families who needed a healing touch and a different approach to their children. Their closeness as friends and similar ways of thinking led to a huge expansion of services around the country as well.

Sudha Kaul (I call her Sudha *mashi*), had been in college with my mother. She wanted to start a school in Calcutta similar to the one in Bombay and began discussing this with mother. I remember a lovely weekend where she, me and mother were all sitting in a large expansive swing together at Ali Bagh (a favourite haunt and get away near Bombay) planning the next school.

Many members of our family were drawn in.

'Midge (a nickname for my mother) what can I do to help?', said my aunt Juniema, over one holiday where she had brought along my cousins.

'Why don't you help someone in Calcutta? Her name is Sudha Kaul', said mother. Together with Sudha *mashi*, and other devoted people, aunt Juniema helped and pioneered the Calcutta Spastics Society.

Then, another person joined us. His name was Sathi Alur and he was a chartered accountant. He first came to the Society to look at its accounts and finances.

'Mithu, I am bringing a finance person to look at our finances', said one of the trustees. Mother, who was always eager for improving the quality of her organization, promptly agreed.

It was 10 February 1978. Wearing a greyish brown safari suit, he walked into mother's office. He had a broad smile, a very open and generous face and was very polite and charming. He spent about 15 minutes looking at the accounts which he felt were in a bit of a mess.

'Well as it so happens, I have got some time to spare as I am between jobs and could help you out', Sathi said. He then asked mother and Pam to conceptualize a five year plan or a vision statement of their dreams for children with disability.

'What is your vision for disabled people in the next five years? What would you like to see if you had the funds?' For mother and Pam, it was a totally novel concept, they had never thought beyond a school.

When Sathi arrived, I was in our drawing room listening to music with my headphones on. He was apparently fascinated by me (so he said later). He had never seen a disabled person, and that too, someone as vociferous as me.

In 1978, another Spastic Society was launched—the Delhi Spastics Society. It was started after an International Conference launched by Mother Teresa and the British Spastics Society. Again, it was begun by a group of friends and two families. Spearheaded by my aunt Mita (*mashi*), and uncle (*mesho*) who had returned from London with a strong desire to serve India and who was now working in AIIMS (All India Institute of

Medical Sciences), a group came together consisting of Anita *mashi*, her husband, uncle Arun (Arun Shourie), and her sister Manju Dubey and Minu *mashi*. My aunt, Radhika, too played a major part.

Now, there were Spastics Societies already in Bombay, Calcutta and Delhi. In 1980, the Spastics Society of Bangalore was set up. Next, the state gave mother five acres of land, and some of her students who had become her good friends, came forward to begin the Spastics Society of Madras. Many people who had known us in England came forward to help. One such person was Leslie Gardner (who I called uncle Leslie). He was the Principal Psychologist at the UK Spastics Society. He had met mother at a conference at University College, Oxford, and offered his services. He visited us three times a year through the British Council, and together with mother, set up the first teacher training course in Bombay. This enabled the beginning of the training of the much needed manpower. The training of teachers began on a national level. All the services set up at that time, in different regions were started either by my mother's students or close members of the family. This is how the five metropolitan cities in India—Bombay, Calcutta, Delhi, Madras and Bangalore—got covered. Mother brilliantly moved away from a centralized to a decentralized model of service, giving help and support wherever needed.

Since Sathi was working, it was only in the evenings that the administrative and finance related works of the organization could be done. Mother, Pam and Sathi worked on the expansion of services after school hours at home, and this became the pattern. After finishing the work, Sathi would want to take us out for treats. He was very affectionate towards us. He knew that there was no father around (I describe this painful period of my life in the next chapter, but my parents separated and eventually went through a divorce). Sathi began to come over on weekends and slowly got to know Nikhil and me. He began to love us and we became extremely close. All of us would go out together like a family.

He fell in love with mother.

After about a year of courting and being the hot favourite with us (we used to tease him later that he probably planned his moves), Sathi proposed to mother. He was warm, affectionate and spiritually inclined; essentially, the healing touch she needed. It was a very romantic time for her. He proposed marriage and she accepted. In 1981, mum and Sathi got married and we became a family again. Their wedding was beautiful, quiet and small, but a well attended affair.

However, while our personal and family lives moved into a happy new chapter, not all was well on other fronts.

I have mentioned the Centre for Special Education earlier in this chapter. I studied in the Centre for eight years and unfortunately, I suffered.

Education in the Centre for Special Education was ad hoc and a little unsystematic. There was no syllabus to follow as they considered themselves to be very liberated educationists. They developed the curriculum in a broad style involving teaching, reading and writing in new methods. We were really the guinea pigs, as educating children with our type of multiple disabilities was all new to them. They saw it to be a very innovative experiment which it was I guess.

We were considered brilliant students. Everything we did was special. We were perceived as a new breed of people who were praised for whatever we did. 'Excellent', 'Very good girl … how well you have done', were the expressions I grew up with. Nobody challenged us. The teachers were happy with one sentence and did not encourage narratives.

This style of education seriously hampered my intellectual growth. I realized later that they did not have a yardstick for achievement, as we were the first children with multiple disabilities to be educated.

'Look at this Mithu, Malini only wrote four sentences on the industrial revolution, and she has been given a very good tick', said dad (Sathi) while teaching me one day.

It is easy for a person with communication problems to pretend that she has learnt something.

'Can you please read this sentence?', dad said as he was tutouring me on my Hindi. I pretended I knew it all and began bluffing my way through. My poor speech had in fact always helped me with my teachers, so why then was he being so difficult? In those days, there were no English or Hindi electronic typewriters to see if we had understood.

I did not have the chance to chatter like normal children did. I had a major communication problem. Was it entirely my fault, or should part of the blame be put on a teacher for not questioning me and making sure I was learning and understanding? The question of course is debatable. Being dysarthric (a medical term to describe people like me who have slow monosyllabic speech), it takes longer for people like me to communicate. We need sympathetic listening, people who will give us a chance to speak out. Not having people who understood me completely did not help. I was imprisoned in my thoughts and did not get the full opportunity to communicate.

Anyone who did not know about my speech problem would think of me as an infant.

Reflecting back on school days, my communication needs were not addressed until I was 13, which is when I was given a Canon Communicator. I began to use it to achieve two-way communication. The Canon Communicator is a small communication aid, the size of a calculator, where my words would come out on a strip of paper, which could be torn off and handed over to a listener.

For me, using it was tedious and I preferred having an interpreter as it speeded things up. Using the Canon Communicator was laborious and much slower than my poor speech. I found it cumbersome as it needed a great deal of effort. It also attracted too much attention. It was terrific for that age and it was slow.

I was lucky in a funny sort of way. I was in the company of adults most of the time. Yes, I was fed and cared for by my family, but where was my intellectual stimulation to come from? I had a close circuit of people who thought I was the cat's whiskers, but where was the scope for improvement? Academically, this had a serious impact on my writing and communication. I did not have any friends in school. We were not taught to mingle. If you have a speech problem, it is equally hard to converse and have an intellectual interaction. My mother boils it down to the diverse backgrounds the students and I came from. Yes, it could be, but it is also true that if individuals have problems of speech, they are less likely to interact. Now with the invention of the internet, people with poor speech can interact easily. My cousins were my only friends from my own generation.

Reflecting on it now, the school was too overprotected and life was over cushioned. A bit of a disaster initially, the school has since then made solid progress. Being trapped in a segregated environment was harmful. If I was in a normal school, I would have seen my normal peers interact. That would have encouraged me and given me a head start on how to be independent in my communication. There is this worldwide debate about whether children with severe disability should be exposed to the normal world? Some professionals believe that it would be better if the child is sheltered in a special school where his/her daily living needs are met. But I question this from my own experience. I feel that if there is no exposure to the outside world, how will any child develop later if he/she is sheltered? The disabled child will naturally imitate what he/she sees. I strongly feel that if the child is exposed to a normal environment from a young age, then the child, however severely disabled he/she is, would have a chance to be included and perhaps accepted by his or her peers and would use his/her own intelligence and social networking skills to develop.

I feel that being trapped in a special school was detrimental to my education. If I did not have my mother who always pushed me, and my entire family who always challenged me, I would not be alive intellectually or physically to tell this tale. I have always felt that this time was the darkest period of my life.

The End of the Beginning

I describe the next eight years as the darkest period of my life. The move back to India was both an end and a beginning. It was the beginning of the Spastics Society but the end of my family.

My parents' marriage broke up. How and why did this happen?

My assessment is that both my parents were involved in initiating something new for the country. My father, using the new expertise he had imbibed as the Director of Gallop Poll in London, was very eager to set up Market Research as a critical need before the launch of products or events. He set up the first Market Research Bureau and called it the Indian Market Research Bureau which was attached to one of the largest Advertising Agencies, J. Walter Thompson, then known as Hindustan Thompson.

Setting up services in a virgin territory, I am sure, was not easy for either of them.

When one is pioneering services in a country, one has to work round the clock. The result was that my parents did not have much time for each other. Each wanted their own separate space. The services completely absorbed and engulfed my mother, and despite his western education, my father appeared to be a fairly traditional man. He wanted more of my mother's time and was not able to accept and cope with this new situation. He wanted my mother to be fresh and ready every evening as being in advertising, my father had to network and socialize often. Having studied child development, my mother was eager to spend all of her free time with my brother and me. She tried really hard to give us some quality time. With all the demands of their work, they did not have time for each other. It also brought home to both my parents, the realization that they were not suited to each other and incompatible in many ways. The result was a divorce.

It is said that parents of disabled children often break up, but in my parent's case I think that as both were so engrossed and involved in work, the conflict of interest was a huge factor that contributed to the breakdown of their relationship, and culminated in a divorce. This was followed by a very traumatic period (again from what my mother relates) for the three of us. I was eight years old and my brother three, when their marriage broke. We couldn't really understand what was happening and why was it happening at all.

Leaving *kaka* (dad) and our big flat in Meherina, where we had been living, was painful. As we left Meherina, I remembered all the good times I had with him. Leaving Meherina also meant leaving our friends. We had many friends in the building and we lost touch with them. Perhaps, if we had stayed on there, my life would have been very different. I would have grown-up with normal friends of my own age.

Mother carried on as if nothing had happened, when actually our life had broken into two. I think she cried silently within. My mother's background helped her; she was brave enough to move away with two children and soldier through life. It was a hard period for my father as well. His family had suddenly gone and he was alone. Divorce was still seen as a taboo in Bombay at that time.

In many ways, it empowered the three of us. My mother called us her soldiers, able to battle and fight. She became greatly empowered through her work and became more independent and assertive.

Our home, which was familiar and comforting for us, was no longer there. When we left Meherina, we left our home, our security nest and most of all, our parents were separated. However much they said that their divorce was amicable, the break-up of any home is hugely traumatic. My parents did everything to keep the pain away from each other, for the sake of the children, but my mother always told us that 'a divorce is a divorce and is always painful and challenging'. It was sad. It was very hard on her and the two of us. Nicky used to ask often 'Where is my Daddy?' I remember the day vividly as we drove down Malabar Hill. Mother was crying as we gave *kaka* a hug. Seeing her, I too started crying. We both cried all the way as we drove to school.

My father stayed in our earlier flat. He remarried a wonderful person named Margot Raymond. During our childhood, we visited our father and Margot once a week.

Looking back on my return to Bombay, it was a lonely existence with no friends, no interaction with children of my age and no school to go to. My brother, Nicky, got admitted to one of the elite private schools but I had nowhere to go. Inclusive Education was a concept which had not yet developed and my mother did not even consider asking this elite school to admit me.

A Family with No Bounds?

Although I had no friends, my cousins were, and still remain, my close friends. Most of my best childhood memories include them. Mother has a brother and a sister. We are six cousins from my mother's side. Her brother Tutu (whom I called Tutu *mama*; *mama* is a term used for mother's brother) married Junie (Juniema), who was mother's best friend from the age of four. Mother and Juniema were inseparable. Juniema and Tutu *mama* had two daughters, Shonali (whom we called Nani or Chonks) and Atiya (we called her Tipla or Tips). Her sister Mita, whom I called *mashi*, married Samiran (I called him *mesho*). I grew up with them in Cambridge and they had a boy Surojit and a girl, Karuna. Karuna was the baby of the family. *Mashi* and *mesho* had her much later, after they came back to India, which was about the same time we came back. Our grandparents *ammi* and *barra dada* kept us all together. I spent a great deal of time with Juniema and *mashi*. They were my surrogate mothers. My father had two sisters, Achla and Pappu. Achla was in New York. She was a teacher and had finished her higher education in Girton College, Cambridge. She has two children, Rahul and Radhika. Pappu and Mahesh have two children, Aditi and Anjali. Nicky and I bonded very well with our cousins. They were like our brothers and sisters. 'Hello Molls', Juniema would say, giving me a kiss, as she took me from mother. As a child, I was always carried. I never felt the need to walk.

My grandparents lived in Bangalore where they had a spacious four bedroom house in Rhenius Street right in the centre of the city. We made regular trips to visit them.

'This is *Babu*', said mother, introducing a good-looking Nepalese gentleman. '*Babu* has been with us since I was a baby', said mother. Mother was born in Darjeeling and *Babu* appeared on the family's doorstep when she was 18 months; he was a young man of 19 at the time. He was brought in by the gardener, who said: 'This man will never leave you.' The gardener was right. *Babu* was trained by *barra dada*. My grandfather loved giving fabulous parties; he adeptly trained *Babu* to make 32 different cocktails. He was polished to become a true British Raj butler of the colonial style. He served as a butler in my grandparents' house for 70 years.

I always enjoyed games with my cousins and they made all efforts to include me. They usually spent their entire long summer holidays with me and Nicky. Although it took Chonks and Atiya a few days to understand my speech, my disability seemed invisible when I was with them. Perhaps, I was cosseted but I feel I was also treated normally by my family. Yes, I was overprotected from the outside world (or as I say, insulated), but whether that was a good thing or bad remains debatable.

'Molls (my pet name), lets imitate the oldies', said Chonks. When we were a bit older, Chonks and I used to spend hours listening to our mothers' gossip. My grandparents' house was huge. My grandfather had his own room tucked at the far end, removed from us by a corridor. As a special treat we would be invited to his room and be given nuts, chips and coke. There was a huge dining room and drawing room. Bangalore was filled with monkeys. A familiar sight in the house was monkeys. Bold and pushy, they were frequently on our dining table.

'There were seven bananas here, where are they?', asked Juniema.

'The monkeys have eaten them', I said, hearing which Juniema laughed. 'That's crazy. Let's close the windows for god's sake!'

As time went on, Chonks had her own set of boyfriends. I did not seem to mind. I was blissfully happy in my segregated set up, giving little thought to boyfriends or the real world. As a child, I had very little contact with the outside world and did not really know the significance of having a boyfriend. Life was beautiful! My family enveloped me with love and shut out the hostile and unfriendly world.

'Remember you young upstarts, don't be enamored by the West; the West is not the best. You must always come back to your own country. I was forced by your aunt', said *mesho* (my uncle Sam) to Nikhil, Suro (Surojit, my cousin) and me. The grown-ups spent an exceeding amount of time with us. Looking back, our relationship with the older generation was like a friendship.

'Have you heard *mesho*?', said mother, trying to sound stern. The family was hugely patriotic, although I personally love England. I remember long dinner table discussions where the importance of serving one's own country was stressed on. *Mesho* loved spending hours chatting with and advising us. All my aunts and uncles spent a huge amount of time with us. We were all made to believe that 'the West is not the Best'. It was a new independent India. Learn the best practices from the West and contribute to India, was a constant advice.

Mother, Juniema, *mashi* and *mama* were involved in setting-up services around the country. As I mentioned earlier, my aunt Juniema helped begin the next special school in the country for children with Cerebral Palsy together with Sudha Kaul in Calcutta. My *mashi* (Mita) helped begin the Centre in Delhi, with Anita Shourie, Manju Dubey, Radhika Roy, Minu Jalan and others. Both centres were aided by mother and developed on the same lines as the first model.

While I was studying in St. Xaviers (more about this in 'Why Do You Want to Do the BA?'), I used to spend every Diwali in Delhi. It was at this time that I started lecturing the disabled students and teachers who worked in the Delhi school at the time.

'Come on Malini, come with me and talk to some of the students in my school', said *mashi*, one day.

'Okay', I said, reluctantly tearing myself away from my romantic novels.

Juniema pioneered and worked in the Spastics Society in Calcutta till she remarried (she too had a divorce) and moved to Bombay.

'Midge can I join you?', asked Juniema when she arrived in Bombay. 'Your help will be invaluable', responded mother, and it was. Juniema was such a special person. She believed that assisting disabled people and children was akin to nectar for her soul.

Juniema joined the Bombay Spastics Society, and took about a year to completely settle into her new life in Bombay. Very often, as there was no car, she would take the congested train from Bandra to Churchgate, partly hanging out of the crowded compartment.

Mesho got a senior position at the AIIMS, a premier institute in the country. The medical institute provided most of the doctors with accommodation depending on their seniority. *Mesho* was first given an E-type house (the houses were rated according to alphabets).

'Hi folks, welcome to our E 78', said *mashi*. *Mashi* had a natural aptitude for interior decoration. She put flowers in the most unlikely places making it look more homely. She was able to make the most of all places she lived in; once she put up a lovely table, covered with a tablecloth and adorned with a vase of flowers, inside a tent in the Loire valley where we were camping.

There is an abrupt jump from the description of the family to a specific instance of a holiday in Kashmir. To better link the two, perhaps a line could be inserted here, which could be read along the lines of—being a very close family, we made every effort to see each other as often as possible. The desire to spend time together encouraged us to plan a family vacation to Srinagar.

My holiday in Kashmir was one of the most unforgettable holidays I have ever had. Me and Nicky accompanied my grandparents, *mesho*, *mashi*, their children (Surojit and Karuna) and Shonali to Srinagar.

Karuna was 11. Nicky and Suro were both 16. Shonali and I were in our early twenties. Our favourite time of day was the afternoon, when we played monopoly. The game was always played like a battle being fought. Fights occurred every five minutes, mainly between Koru and the boys. The boys found great amusement in teasing Koru. Koru would invariably go and tattle on them to her mother.

'When will you grow up?', I chided the boys, 'why do you constantly make Koru cry?'

'Because it's fun' was their response. I returned to my novels feeling disgustingly irritated with them. I wondered when they would finally grow up. The boys were the best of friends, but when it came to which city was better (Delhi or Bombay), they came to fisticuffs.

Mesho would often join them when he was tired of reading Tolstoy's *War and Peace*. During this holiday, *mesho* beat the boys at games like golf and cricket, but this did not destroy their confidence in themselves in the least. They were rather overconfident and full of themselves.

'What shall we do for *dada's* birthday girls?', *Mashi* asked Shonali and me.

'Why don't we ask him?', Shonali replied.

The next day we asked *dada*.

'I have a great desire of celebrating it on the Dal Lake on a houseboat', said *dada*.

'Sounds good to me', said *mashi*, 'what do the rest of you think?'

Ours was a democratic family, where decision making was not a strong point. Collective opinions prevailed and consensual decision making was the order of the day.

Everybody agreed. It sounded like a perfectly good thing to do on one's birthday. A delicious Kashmiri lunch on a houseboat it was to be.

'We can go to MG Road (centre of Srinagar) and finish our shopping', I suggested.

'Yes what a good idea. It will save us one extra trip', said Shonali, a very thrifty person, prudent about expenditure. It was decided that Sam and the children would go ahead and a taxi be arranged for the elders.

On *dada's* birthday, the family got up early. *Mesho* and the five of us walked down the long and winding road. The boys took turns to push my wheelchair. What we did not envisage was the pouring, pelting rain and knee-deep floods at the end of the shopping road. Once the rain began, the wheelchair was impossible to push, despite the boys' efforts at manoeuvring it. Shonali and Koru decided to go ahead towards the lake. 'I told all of you that the wheelchair won't go', laughed Sam. Just then, *mashi, dada, ammi, Babu* and Bingo surfaced and whizzed past us in a white ambassador, completely ignoring us, inadvertently I am sure. They were immersed in their own conversation. The taxi zoomed past the boys, who were now having a tough time experimenting with ways to steer the wheelchair. Eventually, after much waving and screaming, they managed to stop the car. However, even our loud voices were not enough to catch the attention of Shonali and Koru. They were busy gossiping and were not paying attention, due to which we got into the car and only later realized that they were not with us. The boys were then instructed to find the two girls and bring them to a hotel that we spied nearby.

What a mess! It took a long time for them to reach us. The four of them ambled towards us, acting as if time was endless. The girls came first, as the boys were merrily playing some game that they had invented as they strolled along.

When they finally got to us, the grown-ups were seething with rage but managed to keep calm.

'Where have you been? What took you so long? We are starving', said *mashi*, looking very angry. They did not have much to say in defence of themselves.

The usual time for lunch was around 1 o'clock for most people; this family, however, wanted to gorge on authentic Kashmiri food from a top restaurant in Srinagar, regardless of the time of day. It was decided that *mashi* and our grandparents would go to MG Road and buy the food from this restaurant. The rest of the crowd was to stay, put in the lobby of the three-star hotel overlooking the Dal Lake that was serving as our transit home. They thought this would be the ideal waiting place for just half an hour.

Meanwhile, Shonali and I decided that this was the time for a quick shopping trip, as we were leaving for Delhi in four days. We decided to break away from the group and go with the elders, fitting in a round of urgent shopping while they got the food. Everyone had to be pleased in this family!

'I can't take all of you, and see to everyone's needs. It is *dada's* birthday and the time is 1.50 pm. You organize it if you want to. You can follow us, then I can help you too', *mashi* told Shonali.

So off we went. I looked pleadingly at Shonali to take me and she did. She knew that if we did not manage to go today, she would have missed out on her chance of buying anything from Srinagar.

'Okay, let's go', exclaimed Shonali with a spurt of energy.

'Can I come too?', asked Koru, who always wanted to be included with the older girls.

'Okay, if you promise to behave yourself', agreed Shonali.

The group splintered into three. One was left in the hotel, another went to pick up the take away lunch and one went to shop.

We piled into an auto. The wheelchair was folded and kept at our feet. The auto driver was instructed to follow the ambassador but the traffic was maddening, and soon we lost sight of the white ambassador. Koru started whining as she thought she had lost her mum.

'We shall leave you here if you whine', threatened Shonali, which promptly put a stop to the whining. Koru naturally wanted to be with the girls as we were much nicer to her than the boys.

We got down at MG Road, looking totally lost. We looked everywhere for our grandparents and aunt or mother, but they were nowhere in sight. This did not deter us from shopping and we finished it in 45 minutes.

'We must dash, your mum is going to be furious with us', said Shonali.

We arrived looking extremely sheepish, only to find the four men and Bingo standing and waiting patiently out on the road, as the porch of the hotel was flooded to the point that it was impossible to walk through it. Their faces were forlorn and be-reft. I must say, *mesho* was extremely good-natured. The time was 3 pm. Lunch was definitely over for most families.

An hour later, *mashi* and our grandparents returned with bags full of Kashmiri delights, apologizing profusely to us. We jumped onto two Shikaras. Luckily, no one fell into the lake and we ate a mouth-watering lunch, which was unforget-table. However, all of us vowed never to go on a family holiday again!

Boarding School Life—Ugh!

I had studied for eight years at the Centre and the years were hard as I struggled with learning and absorbing the knowledge that was imparted.

I was now 15. It was 1981. It was then that an opportunity to go back to England presented itself.

'Malini should go to Thomas Delarue', said Uncle Leslie one day. 'It is a secondary special school, which the UK Spastics Society runs for bright A-level students, many of whom go on to read for a University degree.'

'Do you want to go to boarding school?', mother asked.

For a year, I mulled over it. My impressions of boarding school were formed by what I had read in adaptations of *Jane Eyre* and Lowood. These books painted a picture portraying life in boarding schools as dismal and cruel.

In 1981, we were to go to London for the summer. I was put onto a wheelchair. This was new for me. Initially, I hated being on a wheelchair because I felt disabled, but I was; when I was young I was never taught to value my disability. The charity model predominated and I was fixed and expected to fit in a round peg hole. If one was disabled, it was expected of him or her to overcome their disability and fit into the able world. This is an oppression that continues till today.

However, once I was on a wheelchair, I loved it. I was back in my favourite place, my second home, London. I visited all the famous sites of London with my family and friends: Trafalgar Square, Madame Tussauds, all the national galleries and parks. We spent an endless amount of time just hanging around and imbibing the atmosphere in London. We all agreed with my grandfather, who too loved London, when quoting Ben Johnson, he said, 'he who is tired of London is tired of Life'.

'We are going to visit Thomas Delarue next week. Would you like to spend the night there?', mother asked, always being democratic.

'Yes, why not?', I said quite eagerly.

When we arrived at the Thomas Delarue School, mother and uncle Leslie showed me around the premises. The headmaster greeted us in a clipped Oxonian accent. The school was spread over five acres of land which had been gifted by a philanthropist. The school building sprawled over two acres (the largest school building we had ever seen) and the gardens and lawns were undulating over three acres. The school was fully accessible and wheelchair friendly. There were several classrooms, a science lab and an art room. Additionally, there were two therapy rooms with physiotherapists—an occupational therapy room and a speech therapy room. The school also had a large, beautiful hall, the centre-piece of which was a piano that was supposed to be the Spastics Society's showpiece. The school had four dormitories.

My one night and day at the school were pleasant. We were put to bed at 8.30 pm and woken up at 7 in the morning. I noticed that even those with the severest disabilities were extremely independent. I slept with three girls. They were friendly and welcoming.

'How was your night?', asked mother and uncle Leslie, being very inquisitive.

'Would you like to come and study here?', uncle Leslie asked.

'Perhaps', I said, cuddling up to mother. I felt unsure and at that point I did not want to think about leaving mother. But I pondered over it and realized that things were too stagnant in Bombay. In school, we were not being challenged. There were no formal exams. The Centre for Special Education had not yet had any student sitting the Board exams. Ironically, after I left, three of my class mates did the Secondary School Certificate (SSC) which made them eligible to go to college. I was bored by the monotony of life in Bombay. The education offered was not challenging enough and the negative attitude of people to-wards me made me and mother very despondent.

'Shall I go?', I asked Shonali.

'Yes you should go, even I am going to boarding school next year', she said. I always needed someone my own age to consult when making a difficult decision. When I was young, owing to my slow speech, family members were under the impression that I was overly dependent on mother. Little did they know that despite my poor speech, I had a definite mind of my own, though due to lack of exposure and perhaps, a lack of indepen-dent movement, the mind was uncertain and hazy. I wanted to try out something different, something new. I felt I needed a change.

I decided three months later that I would take the plunge of moving away from home and mother and enrol at boarding school.

'I want to go to Delarue', I finally said to mother.

'A good idea', said uncle Leslie and began the process of trying to get a scholarship for me.

At that time, Tim Yeo was the Chairman of the Spastics Society of UK. As uncle Leslie was Principal Psychologist of the Spastics Society of UK, the Indian link with the British Society was strong. I got a scholarship from the Society. Neither of my parents were earning in pounds anymore and the tuition fee would have been a huge expense for us. Thus, the scholarship helped tremendously.

It was the end of August when we landed at Heathrow. Goodbyes were hard for me. I howled all through immigration. It was tough when I had to say bye to mother.

They left me on a Sunday evening. I was very sad to part with them and cried my heart out. One would have thought that over the years I would become stronger, but no such luck. To this day, I am an embarrassment when I cry. I bawl loudly. One of my many handicaps, I guess.

Delarue, along with most British schools, started its new academic year early September. Our daily routine began at 7 am. Most of us were in deep sleep and rarely heard the bell. Sometimes, I would get up before the bell and have a bit of time to myself before the other students woke up. Delarue was short of care staff and we had to do most of the things ourselves. For me, this was difficult as in India, everything was done for me. For instance, I had never made my bed; there was always someone there to make it for me. It was a different experience for me.

I learnt by watching other disabled girls all trying to do what they could. As part of the school curriculum, we went to the occupational therapist once a week. She showed us the best way to take our clothes off and put them back on. I was slow and found it a huge effort.

Breakfast was served at 8 am on weekdays. On Saturdays, we were given an extra hour. Saturdays were free and I spent the morning doing the pending homework. Dinner was at 6 pm, which was frightfully early for me. I was not accustomed to eating so early so I ended up filling my stomach with chocolates. I used to drown my sorrow of being so far away from home by eating lots of chocolates.

Most of us were bright and followed a set curriculum. The school functioned like a normal secondary school with all subjects being taught. Academics were hard for me at Delarue. The others had an edge over me as they had all gone to formal schools. It was clear that I had not received much of a formal education. My subjects were geography, science, maths, history and english.

I liked english and enjoyed writing essays. However, I struggled with writing narratives. My geography teacher was extremely good looking. Instead of focusing on geography, we concentrated on his good looks. My history teacher, Mr Lacy, had served in the Indian army. Often, we did not quite understand what he was saying as he spoke with a nasal accent. Mr Lacy spoke to me in a smattering of hindi, which I barely understood. His accent used to keep me in splits. I had to control myself from bursting out laughing. I was hopeless in science as I had not been exposed to it before coming to Delarue.

'Malini does not have a brain for science', said the science teacher to my mother. I was beginning to feel I had no brain at all. I was poor in science and geography.

The school finished at 4 pm. The teachers dispersed immediately. We watched them in our wheelchairs and crutches as they toddled off home and we remained imprisoned in the school.

One year, when England had her worst winter, Delarue was snowbound.

'I am sorry, but the pipes are frozen', said the headmaster at the morning assembly. 'You have two weeks off.' I went to Wimbledon to live with uncle Leslie and his wife Mary, who were my local guardians. They took care of my needs. My friend Amena, who had come down to Wimbledon from India, also helped. I still remember that once Amena was pushing me up the hill on a cold, winter day. Amena had a very mild balancing problem because of which she had a particular gait (somewhat like a drunken sailor). We had accepted her peculiar walk as a normal part of her. To balance herself while walking, she would sway from side to side. As we were walking down Wimbledon Common, we were stopped by a policeman who was clearly not used to people swaying from side to side unless they were drunk.

'Stop', instructed the policeman. He thought Amena was drunk because of her ataxic gait and wanted to breathalyze her. Only after speaking to her did he realize that she was not drunk, lived nearby and he let her go. Amena is most capable and a very organized a person. Poor Amena, what an experience it must be not being able to walk like everyone else.

One day, when in class at Delarue, some of the students and I were yanked out of school at an unearthly hour in the morning to meet the Indian Prime Minister, Indira Gandhi, who was visiting London. We had to wear our uniform and I was selected to give her a clock as a small token. She was very sweet to me. I remember the young Sonia Gandhi was accompanying her. They had come to inaugurate an exhibition organized by the Spastics Society of India (Bombay).

One day I discovered everyone getting ready to go shopping.

'Where are they going?', I asked my housemother, Pam. Everyone in Delarue had one house parent. The girls and the younger boys had housemothers and the older boys had housefathers. Pam was from the south of England and was extremely prim and proper. Pam wanted to make us all completely English. 'They are going shopping', she said.

'Why can't I go?', I asked.

'You have to sign your name on a sheet that is stuck next to the library if you wish to go.' I liked Pam but she wanted me to be more and more organized. I was disappointed but promised to be sharper next time, so as to not miss out on the opportunity for various trips.

I quickly learnt to better organize my time. I put my name down early on Wednesday for the shopping trip and for a trip to the post office.

Once when I picked up the sausage with my fingers, Pam made me put down my sausage and cut it up, thrusting a fork in my hand. 'Malini, this is not the way to eat sausages. We eat it with a knife and fork', said Pam.

During my first year at school, I had a manual wheelchair that I would push with my feet. It was bad for my posture as I had to push my wheelchair backwards. The Delarue physiotherapists argued with my mother, insisting that this practice was good for my independence. One day I fell and nearly broke my nose. My mother was horrified and made a big fuss and complained. It was then that I was permitted to have an electric wheelchair.

With my electric wheelchair, I was extremely mobile. For the first time, I could move with ease anywhere I liked.

Who cared if I could not walk? With an electric wheelchair I could run. For the first few days I used the chair sparingly but once I became familiar with using the joystick, I went everywhere. It was absolutely fabulous. For the first time I could move large distances unassisted. I was not dependent on anyone.

Although I did not like the structure and the regimentation of life, Delarue taught me to grow up and be responsible for myself. It taught me to be assertive about my needs, organize my time, and in a sense it prepared me for a regular college like St. Xavier's College in Bombay. It was hard, but after two years, I got my General Certificate for Secondary Education which made me eligible to get into St. Xavier's.

As Abraham Lincoln had said to his son, who was studying in a boarding school, 'The best steel goes through fire.' Only, I was not the best steel.

Two
GROWING UP

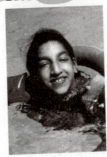

Why Do You Want to Do the BA?

I was admitted to St. Xavier's Junior College, Bombay, one of the most prestigious colleges in India, to do my Higher Secondary Certificate (HSC), which is a two-year pre-university programme (it can be compared to the 'A' levels in England, though certainly not on par). It was the first time that I was going to come in contact with a mass of normal students. Would I be accepted socially? Would I be able to cope academically?

Initially, there was some trouble as people did not have the experience or education about people with disability.

'Why do these students want to give this exam?', was the response of the Vice Chancellor of Bombay University, to a request by mother and Pam that the university make available the option of extra time for disabled students sitting in an exam.

'These exams are a waste of time. They are useless, and these students would be better kept at home', she said.

Mother had by then managed to create much needed awareness about my condition. When she began her discussions with the authorities, they were very open to listening to her. She was promised all forms of support by the authorities. Mother argued valiantly for certain demands, and eventually succeeded in having them addressed.

Along with me, there were three other students from the Centre for Special Education who had taken the school leaving exam or the Secondary School Certificate (SSC), which is recognized by the Maharashtra State Board. I had completed the GCSE at Delarue which was considered an equivalent. The four of us—Bharat Shah, Farhan Contractor, Andrea Row and I—were the first students with multiple disabilities to enrol at a mainstream college in India. We created history by making the concept of inclusive education in higher education, a reality in India for the first time.

St. Xavier's College was founded in 1869 by German Jesuits, and was named after the Roman Catholic Missionary St. Francis Xavier. It was situated right in the centre of the city of Bombay close to the Victoria Terminus. As one entered, there was a porch and a small decorative garden, leading to a reception where students or staff could get information and make phone calls. One then approached the first quadrangle (popularly known as the first quad) where students would sit under the arches and while away the hours. The auditorium divided the first quad from the second. One could sit in the second quad, but, as it was close to the canteen, it got very noisy and was not as comfortable. The canteen was the nerve-centre, the hub of the college. Throngs of students congregated at the canteen at various points of the day. Beyond the canteen were some trees and a hostel for boys, next to which was the residence for the priests.

The main building of the college comprised of four floors. The first floor housed the office and one of the libraries. The second and the third floor were mainly lecture halls. The fourth floor consisted of the living quarters of some of the priests.

There were two lifts. One lift was built in the last century. It had a key which, besides me, only the Fathers kept. I was privileged enough to be given a key enabling me to operate the lift. It was small and my electric wheelchair could just about fit in, but with a great deal of pushing, pulling and adjusting, I would squeeze in. The second lift was at the far end and was a bit bigger. Neither of the two lifts stopped on the mezzanine floor, where the library was situated. This later proved to put me at a great disadvantage. I could never spend much time in the library. The lifts being old, I was dependent on them more than I desired.

A question that I am often asked by journalists is whether I felt as if I was different. I most certainly did. I think it was in Xavier's where the differences hit me.

It was my first day at Xavier's, and I did not know how others were going to react to my disability. I entered the classroom. There was a stunned silence. The silence was interrupted by the irritating, incessant noise of the motor of my electric wheelchair. There were whispers and unsure shuffles. The professor himself looked most scared and apprehensive.

They must have wondered who this heap of undulating mass in an electric wheelchair was. Had she entered the wrong class? I parked myself in the front row. The class began. At least the entrance was over with.

'Your names please', said the professor, turning to the person next to me.

'Malini Chib', I said my name, which I know sounded completely garbled to all around me. No one understood. The professor looked perplexed. He asked again. I spoke again. He thought I had not understood the question. He was irritated, so were 88 other students. I tried spelling my name. He did not get me. I began to panic. I tried again. My speech was getting worse and worse. He looked away impatiently. He had not understood. I heard a cry from a student from behind. 'She said "Malini"'. Eureka! She had understood at last. I had held up the class for 15 minutes. The professor smiled reluctantly but I did not care. At least I had overcome the first hurdle. Now, 88 of my classmates knew my name. They also knew that I had a speech problem. Although it was awful to have all those piercing eyes staring at me, I was happier than before I came in. Now I had some identity. I was not just a lump of flesh on a wheelchair.

This exercise was repeated five times during the day as each lecturer wanted to know the names of their students. By the third lecture, some of the students had befriended me, and they said my name for me, which I liked because it was quick and not so embarrassing. My name pronounced and spoken properly sounded much nicer than my own speech, which tends to be a kind of a monotone.

Another hurdle was that both my tools of communication, namely, my speech and hand function, were damaged. I could not write with a pencil and could not take down notes. I mostly used a typewriter, as in those days computers were rare. Mother came up with a new method. She gave my classmates a pad with a sheet of carbon paper. This way the lectures could be covered and I would be given a copy. I depended on them for my notes, which were important as the textbooks did not go into too much detail. My classmates seemed to like doing the task for me. For answering questions in class, I used a Cannon Communicator.

To my surprise, often the students were not bothered with what the lecturer had to say, as they were busy mindlessly chattering amongst themselves. I could not participate with them as my speech was not loud enough and no one understood me clearly. I used to type what I wanted to say on the Cannon. My speech was slow and laborious, yet what could I do? I had so much to say but I could not contribute quickly. I felt left out, isolated and frustrated at not being able to participate and contribute to conversations fast, like my normal peers. Previously, I was in special schools, where life was at a slower pace. Professionals and others were trained to listen to all of us sympathetically and they would give that extra time we needed to get across what we wanted to say.

Break time for me was not a normal event. It was a huge obstacle, as far as accessibility was concerned. I had to be physically helped. I was taken by a few girlfriends to one of the lifts. We had to barge into classroom after classroom as the lift was at the other end of the corridor, which ran through all the classrooms. Although I used an electric wheelchair, I needed help as there were ledges at the end of each classroom acting as barriers curtailing my independence. I was different and obviously I needed help with these barriers. What an absurd architect. Why do all normal people think that everyone in the world must keep to the norm of the walking pattern, and if one does not walk like everyone else, one will be left out of life? As I passed each classroom, the lecturer would stop speaking, and the whole class' attention would turn towards me, until I passed through. It was terribly painful being the cynosure of all watchful eyes and those few minutes always seemed like an agony.

Owing to extreme problems of physical accessibility and due to my limitations with quick speech, I could foresee that I was going to have problems.

The most important activity in college was socializing. It was the first time I had mingled with people my own age. Would people understand me? Would they feel embarrassed talking to me? Were they coming up to me just because I was disabled? For the first few weeks I zoomed around saying hello to a couple of people whom I knew. Generally however, I moved about on my own as I felt shy to initiate a conversation. Although I had friends who were normal, I used to always meet them individually. I soon found out, painfully, that my vocal expression was not quick enough to be included in a dynamic interactive group situation. This was another agonizing experience. No effort was made by those who could speak. My speech became my biggest barrier. Again the same formula dominated all these normal people—anybody not speaking like everyone else would literally be rejected and abandoned.

It took me a long time to come to terms with it. I began questioning myself. Did I have my own personality? Was I just another disabled girl who needed things done for her? I knew that I was different and trapped in a dysfunctional body, but did others realize I had a spirit and a mind separate from this body? My body did not work like others, but did they realize that my mind was normal? Did they consider thinking that my desires were just the same as theirs?

Socially therefore, life was hard. I was coming from a background of having studied at a special school in England. All the others had already met up with their peers; a majority of students were from various schools in Bombay, so most had some friends and belonged to some group or gang.

I began to feel that just like my dysfunctional body, my mind was also dysfunctional. I could also never think like them. I began doubting myself and my abilities.

It was not a good beginning, but I eventually realized that I must be determined to fight. I would show them that, except for my body, I was just like them. I was not going to give up.

'Let's go to a movie', said Feroza, a girl from my class. I had just joined them after my wanderings. 'Yes, which one?', Khushid asked. 'Why not *Kramer vs. Kramer* or *An Officer and a Gentleman*', suggested Pervez. 'Yes, why not?' 'It's 12 o'clock, and if we hurry we can make it for the 1 o'clock show', said Khushid. The gang was informed. I was automatically left out. All I had to do was to tell them how to handle me, but I was not fast enough or pushy enough, and everything was organized very quickly. I, obviously, was going to be a problem for them, so it was just easier to leave me out. They must have assumed that I have no feelings and, thus, how could I feel left out?

I went up to class feeling hurt. I wanted them to make that extra bit of effort, but they were not prepared to do so in what seemed to me a thoughtless, mindless pursuit of enjoyment.

Nevertheless, one day I did make it to a movie with them because I was determined to invite myself, so I opened the subject and asked my gang of friends if we could go for a movie. I wanted to show them that I too could go to the cinema. 'Yes why not?', they said a little doubtfully. 'I can walk if two people hold me on either side, under the arm', I suggested enthusiastically. They were caught up with the enthusiasm of the novelty of it and agreed. 'We'll take my car', I said. We went and saw *The Champ* and I managed to walk up the stairs of the New Excelsior with their help. After the movie, we stuffed ourselves with *bhel* and *pani puri* at Vithals. It had been a success. The group had enjoyed my company, and they had not felt that I was a burden on them. It was the first of many outings. Though I generally had to be the first one to initiate and organize these, my friends usually complied readily.

However, the process of normalization proved to be hard because I wanted to be a part of everything around me and often could not be. Dances, picnics, parties—I could not be a part of the normal mainstream of life because of my severe disabilities.

It is then that I began my journey of deep introspection. What is normal? Who is normal? Why am I abnormal? Who decides? I cannot speak, I cannot walk; does that make me abnormal? It seemed obvious that I was different. I began to be painfully aware that I was never going to be easily accepted by so-called normal society.

Academically, I am happy to recollect, I was treated equally with others. My first set of exam results were a dismal failure. 'I have got your unit test papers back', said our English teacher. I thought I had done fairly well but I was mistaken. The papers came rolling in one by one. My marks were abysmally low. I had failed the first unit test. I had performed badly in all my six papers. I felt terrible, defeated and embarrassed, as just when I had made some friends and thought that I had communicated to them that I was intelligent, they saw my results. I was awfully ashamed and felt very small and inadequate.

Mother came to my rescue. She analyzed it all for me and said that it was not because I was not intelligent but because I was not used to the rote kind of learning which was the practice in India. For two years in England, I was trained to conceptualize what I learnt, but here I had to produce answers straight from the book. My mother, as usual, took up the cudgels, and took charge of my education. She diligently tutored me for the next five years.

I learnt that the examiners wanted narrative and essay type of answers. They preferred quantity rather than quality. I gave short multiple choice answers because I had been taught that at Thomas Delarue. Many a time I would not succeed in remembering words exactly as they were in the text book. Also long answers needed a great deal of effort. It was a hard task to master, especially since I had poor speech and poor hands. Our sessions would often end in tears.

'Why can't you understand that what you have told me about the French Revolution is all in your own words?', mother scolded. 'The examiners don't want that. Your English may be perfect, but it won't do for the exam. You have to use the words of the book. Please mug the words up', she said as she handed me the book. She brought me model answers which I chose to reject, because I did not like the English.

There was a lot to remember. I was given double the time, which was four hours. I had a lot to say and wondered if my writer would understand everything I said in what seemed a short span of four hours.

I had to be tutored in Economics and French. The HSC (Higher Secondary Certificate) required the study of a language, the two options available being Advanced Hindi and Basic French. My Hindi was dreadful. I was just about able to communicate with the people who were helping us. I was lucky that Xavier's was offering French as I had not done Hindi, having completed my 'O' levels in England.

I made two close friends in class, namely, Christine and Feroza. Christine was short, dark and a staunch Catholic. She had long, jet black hair which she usually tied into a bun. Feroza was fair, tall and a Parsi. Christine, Feroza and I always sat at the back, discussing the most important part of our lives—our social lives. Studies were the least of our worries. Our chatter usually consisted of when the next party was, or what happened at our last party, or who said what to whom.

I loved these conversations as it would make me feel normal.

'Malini please be quiet', instructed my Economics lecturer. New lecturers did not initially notice the difference in me from the rest of the class, as I had migrated to the back benches. Once they knew that I was disabled, they would come and ask whether I had any difficulty in understanding and said to come to them if I needed any help. It was my second year. I had passed the first year. I was trying very hard to whisper something to Christine. I had by then, gotten accustomed to the behaviour of other students, and used to sit at the back, blabbering away to friends. The Economics lecturer knew my speech well as she was giving me extra help. There were advantages and disadvantages in getting extra help from lecturers.

Another part of college life was boyfriends. There was much time to mingle with boys as classes finished by three in the afternoon. We were a part of a big gang. We all attended the same parties. Feroza was highly popular with the opposite sex. Varun Batra, who was a friend of ours, took a liking to her. He was one of the first few men who actually talked to me.

'Are you ready?', said Feroza, she had come to pick me up, as we were going to yet another party. She had brought a guy from the Doon School. He was cute looking and we nicknamed him Dodo.

'What do you think of him?', Feroza asked me.

'He's cute', I said. That was a mistake because she went and told the rest of the group and tried to pair us off as she thought that I needed a boyfriend. This did not materialize, but we remained good friends.

Mayo, Varun and Rajdeep were the few men who took the trouble to get to know me and understand my speech. Most others looked at me as if I was still a child. It was a combination of their shyness as well as an unsurety about what to do and how to act. I think it also had to do with their 'macho' image. For the typical boy, it was not acceptable to be seen with a disabled girl-friend. They wanted a 'normal girlfriend' on their arm.

Yet I loved the normalcy of life I had at Xavier's.

It was a black Monday when I got a call from Feroza.

'You are also on the blacklist', said Feroza, who sounded quite pleased on the phone.

'I don't believe it. You must be joking', I said.

'No, I am serious, and your percentage of attendance is lower than mine', said Feroza. Students at Xavier's needed 75 per cent attendance. Else, they may not be promoted to the next class.

'How is that possible?', I screeched. 'You were absent more often than me because of Malhar', I said in a confident tone.

Malhar was a college festival that took place every year. All the colleges of Bombay participate in it. The festival usually lasts for three days. Games, quizzes, music contests and debates between colleges were organized. Feroza was selected as the sec-retary of the organizing committee. So we expected her name to come out on the blacklist, but not mine.

I normally attended the first three lectures, the first beginning at 9 in the morning. I was very conscious of being on time otherwise I would interrupt the other classes. It was easier for Feroza as other students could proxy her name and roll number for her. For me it was impossible as I could not be missed by anyone. I stood out like a sore thumb.

'So, Miss Chib, you are on the blacklist, at last', said Sagari and Shahnaz as they sipped their tea. They were good friends who loved to tease me. 'We always knew you would be.'

'Now, what do we have to do?', I said woefully.

'We have to go to the Principal's office and explain why our attendance is low', said Feroza.

I went with Feroza. The Vice Principal looked stern and gave us a long speech about the consequences of missing lectures.

'If your attendance is below 75 per cent, you will not be allowed to sit for the HSC', he said in his heavy South Indian accent. As he rattled on about the consequences, I transfixed my gaze to my navel as I found it difficult to control my laughter. I found his way of speaking very funny. He seemed quite assured that since I was looking down, I was very penitent. We solemnly signed a slip of paper and left. The tension of the previous two days disappeared. We were free to do whatever we liked, but we also knew that we had our responsibilities. After all, we were not in school anymore.

Secretly, I felt normal; I too had been blacklisted like anyone else!

'All the best', I said to Feroza.

It was the night before the HSC exam. We were all ringing up one another to extend good luck wishes. I had been given double the time. It was two hours for my friends but four for me. I could type but my speed was acutely slow. For one question, the answer had to be four pages long and if I were to type, one answer would take me four hours. I needed writers who could understand me and write quickly. People who write for others are known as emanuencies. There was a rule that the emanuencies had to be younger than the student, a rule which suited the visually impaired but which was not conducive to the special needs of people like me who suffered from a speech problem. After much sustained negotiation with officials of the Bombay University, Deepak (Deepak Kalra, Senior Director of the Spastics Society of India, who pioneered training) and Pam managed to get me the provision of double the time and allow the choice of amanuenses to be made by me.

'How was English?', Suzanne, another friend who understood my speech very well, asked me.

'It was okay, except we were in a noisy room and people kept using it as a corridor. It was hard for Pam who was writing for me, to hear what I was saying. But we did manage eventually to get a quiet room for ourselves in Elphinstone College', I said.

Each paper was four hours long. This was just about bearable. The whole process was tedious as I had to regurgitate what I had learnt for four hours at a stretch. Nicky, Sathi, Juniema and Varsha, all wrote for me. I had to be given some water and juice separately. It was also strenuous for those writing for me, in continuously trying to comprehend my monotonous, expressionless speech. I felt that I was just disgorging out the facts, rather than thinking and creating an answer. It has been said frequently, and I agree, that the education system in India teaches students to be like sausage machines rather than thinkers of the future.

As I was isolated at another venue, and finished the exam much later than my peers, I missed meeting my friends after the exam to compare the answers.

The day then arrived when the HSC results were put up on the board.

'Malini has got a first', exclaimed my very excited aunt Juniema over the phone, to mother. We were spending the summer in London.

'So darling, what subjects are you going to do in college for your BA?', Juniema asked, after I passed my HSC.

She read the Xavier's prospectus and told me which subjects were compulsory. I vividly remember her sitting in our drawing room sifting through the Xavier's prospectus, reading it out and discussing it with me. I recollected that when I was young, it was Juniema who was interested in and always encouraging my academic development.

I was supremely happy. For the first time, I was on par with my peers, academically.

I had gotten admission into the degree programme. For my BA, I had originally chosen all six papers in Psychology, but the department, aware of my poor hand function, warned me that Psychology demanded a great many experiments be performed. I changed to a double major in English and Psychology, with History as an ancillary.

Feroza was going to Sorbonne in Paris as her mother had gotten a job with the French Consulate. Christine too was not going to be in the same class as she was doing different subjects.

I had to make new friends all over again. It was not going be easy. I was again left alone. It was as if I was thrown into the deep blue sea, and I could not swim to save my life. I would have to make that effort of proving that I was intelligent again. Fortunately, and surprisingly, it turned out to be easier than my first year at Xavier's.

'We have something in common', said Geeta one day. I was on my own having a drink in the canteen.

'What is it?', I said.

'Both our parents are divorced', said Geeta, who was a Parsi. Geeta was short, fair and was always dressed in trousers or shorts. Geeta was in my English class. There were a couple of new students from Sophia College who seemed to be lost.

The BA classes were different from HSC classes as they were held on the third floor where the lift could not reach. I was helped by my friends, and with two people holding me on either side, I could manage. The indignity of it, the visibility of my disability being pronounced glaringly, was very demeaning. We informed the lecturers and the management about the matter, and tried to make the classes shift to a floor that was accessible by the lift, but they turned a deaf ear and told us that the lecturers themselves wanted their classes in certain rooms. The lecturers, in turn, placed the responsibility with the management. All this was highly complicated and, eventually, we gave up, realizing that our efforts to shift the classroom were futile. There was obviously no proper policy. It was an act of favour and charity to have me there, and they were not going to adjust if it meant the slightest inconvenience.

'There is no point getting you down because in 35 minutes, we've got FC', said Geeta. FC was the short form for Foundation Course that was compulsory in the first year of the BA Programme. It gave us first year students a basic though comprehensive picture of India's social, economic and political history.

A few of us sat in the class and jabbered away the hour. With the use of my Canon Communicator, I was able to make friends with a couple of girls from Sophia College. Carol, a girl who had also done 'O' levels like me, shared with me the difficulty in understanding the English used in the textbooks we were meant to study. The authors who wrote the textbooks used such poor language, which was simplistic and uninspiring. We had to try and make a conscious effort to use beginner's English in essays and exams, rather than engage with complex words and phrases.

Another friend was Tina from Denmark. She had big, dark blue eyes which looked frightening as she would gaze hard at anyone who would stare at us. This happened mostly when Elsa and I were struggling to fit my wheelchair into the narrow lift. Men would stand and stare at us, and it would drive us mad. They would never voluntarily come up and help.

'Oh no, why is this lift so damn small and why do these chauvinist bastards persist on staring rather then helping?' Elsa used swear words freely and I quite liked to hear them, as it would somehow release all the venom in me.

'Indian Male Chauvinistic Bastards!' This was soon abbreviated to our secret code IMCB. So appropriate, I secretly thought.

However, like most women my age, I loved the company of men. I would try and seek them out and initiate a conversation, but unfortunately, the 'poor little bastards' had never been taught to reach out beyond their own needs and so, they did not know what to do with me. Only a handful of men would make that extra bit of an effort to understand my atypical speech. But they never really went beyond superficial chatting.

Social events continued to make me get into dregs of depression because I got the feeling that I was never really wanted.

Two occasions remain in my mind. Prom Night was one of them.

'Are you coming to Prom Night?', Lyla asked Tina.

'No, I have not been asked', said Tina.

'Neither have I', said Lyla, 'let's go in a big gang of girls'. We went like bold women, fully confident that we were going to get partners. The boys were in their one and only formal suits. The girls wore long dresses or mini skirts. There was loud music playing in the background. We got a table and chatted amongst ourselves. We began dancing in a group. I danced with my crutches. After a little while one of the organizers came up and said rather patronizingly: 'Why don't you sit down, you are bound to fall. You can't dance with crutches.' Geeta and Tina gave her a dirty look and were furious with her. Human beings were obviously averse to and not used to crutch dancing. I, like a fool, sat down promptly. Slowly my group of friends disintegrated and went to the dance floor joining their men friends.

The fun was over. I was no longer a part of them. I watched them dance and that terrible emotion, which I rarely allow to surface began to assail me. I wondered if there would ever be a man in my life. Would a man see beyond my body? Would anyone put their arms around me and dance with me? Would anyone kiss me passionately? Would I ever be needed by a man emotionally or would I always be regarded as a burden for someone to take care of? A silent tear unseen by any human eye trickled down my face as Lionel Richie's 'Hello' blared in the background, the dancer's put their arms around each other and were lost in discovering each other's world.

I was left alone with my thoughts. The realization that I would be disabled all my life dawned upon me. I had always imagined that when I grew up, I would be normal.

Another occasion I remember was lunch at Nargis' house. It was Nargis' birthday. Her house was small but colourful. The curtains were bright pink and the sofas had floral furnishing. We met Nargis' parents for the first time. They were elderly Parsees. Nargis' mother wore a clean, crisp blue dress, which looked cool to the eye.

'Lunch is served', said her mother. The table was filled with delicious dishes. There was the famous *dhansak*, which was made with four *dals* (lentils); it could be eaten with rice or bread. A salad and two vegetables were served. Not to forget the mouth-watering Bombay-duck which is not a duck, but a fish; it is a Parsi specialty.

I was rather oversensitive about my eating, as I would make a mess all around the side of the plate and my mouth would sometimes be covered with food. Therefore, I always preferred to sit and eat at the table. After serving me, Geeta and Ellen joined the crowd with a plate full of food. The lunch was a buffet.

'Sit here with Molls and have your lunch', said Nargis' mother to Nargis.

'No, I want to sit with my friends and eat', she replied, as if I was not there and could not hear or understand. I would have obviously liked to have eaten with them but it was virtually impossible for me to hold a plate and eat while making polite conversation. I sat and ate in solitude as the others chatted away, quite unaware that I had not been able to join them.

I felt terribly hurt. It was as if I had to be invited and so for courtesy's sake, I was. People did not really want my company. They were oblivious to my needs and could not see my physical difficulties with eating.

It made me question what I wanted from these social gatherings. Why did I go? Was it the food or the company that I went for? It taught me to be a bit distant from my friends, as I seemed to collapse emotionally if they did something which upset me.

My college years threw up new challenges on a variety of fronts—social, personal and academic. I learnt to grapple with these challenges and overcome obstacles thrown in my way.

It was during these years that I lost someone who had played a very important part in my life, who had been the first to encourage me to enrol at college for a higher degree.

For the 42 days that Juniema was sick and was admitted in the Breach Candy hospital, we all practically lived in the hospital and only came home at night. All of us lived in our house. Nicky, Shonali, Tiya (Shonali's sister and my cousin) and I slept on the drawing room floor, while we left the beds for the grown-ups. Juniema was operated upon four times. By the third week she went into a coma.

We lost her on 2 December. It was the most tragic blow that stunned and shocked the whole family. She was only 42.

For me it was losing a friend, mentor and a second mother who had loved and supported me through all my trying times.

I had to get used to life without Juniema, and one way of doing so was to immerse myself into college life and activity so as to temporarily distract myself, and learn to move on with life.

It was the second year of the BA Programme. I had English, Psychology and History. In History, we were studying Modern India, from the period of 1890 to 1960. I loved studying British India and the Indian Independence struggle. In English, we were studying T.S. Eliot. There was also a paper in Mass Communication.

In Psychology we were studying Social Psychology. Some of the topics that we covered were group behaviour. What attracts people? What are the physiological and other factors that transpire when two people meet? What are the chemical reactions that take place between them?

We had Maya Mehta and Uma Pinto, Nicky told us Maya Mehta was taking the class on *Murder in the Cathedral* and Uma Pinto would be teaching us poetry. 'In poetry we are studying Eliot's The Wasteland', said Nicky.

Uma's first lecture left us baffled. She spoke in clipped English. Uma was tall and usually wore white. She would always treat us as some lesser mortals. We nicknamed her the 'white witch' because we took a strong disliking to her. She, of course knew her work, and was proficient in her subject. She spoke with a confident air in her voice. We were all petrified of the way she spoke.

I said, 'I have never found anyone teaching English at Xavier's, who speaks as well as Uma.'

'Yes I like her, but she is a bit uptight and pompous.' Nicky said, 'speaking with an Oxonian accent and behaving in a highly superior manner'. 'Why does she speak in such a condescending way as if we were far below her station in life?' Uma had a knack of pointing her finger at Nicky and asking for her opinion. We had to quietly put up with all her patronizing ways as she was a well-known poet in the city.

Uma handed our terminal exam papers back. We had all failed.

'You are all good for nothing; you will never get through the finals. You will never pass and you will be stuck here all your life, because you don't read enough', she shrieked. 'I wonder, if you use your grey cells at all, or for that matter if you even have any.' Every time we came out we felt completely demoralized. We had to even tolerate her for Mass Communication. She used to insist that we saw the most depressing and macabre films. She usually organized Russian films at the Russian Consulate for us. These films were highly morbid and had Russian subtitles.

'All of you need to study more. You all have to put in at least three hours of reading', she said. 'Now if you only had done all your references and not wasted your time in silly college activities, then you might have passed.' She went on to point out all our common mistakes. While she ranted and raved, I had an involuntary athetoid movement and one arm of my wheelchair flew open, which made a loud clutter and fell on the floor with a big bang. Uma stopped talking for a minute to see what, or who, had caused the noise. All eyes turned towards me. I was deeply embarrassed. She realized what the matter was, ignored it and proceeded with her groaning, but she seemed to have lost the continuity and got very tired of us and dismissed the class early. Many came up to me after the class and congratulated me!

The poem 'The Wasteland' looked highly complicated and confusing. I did not know how I was going to master it. I was convinced that I was going to fail that year.

'You need to do a lot more reference work', Uma repeatedly said in every class. Her words kept echoing in my mind.

How was I going to pass this year? I could not go the library and spend hours like my friends, as the lift did not go there. I wished I could spend time studying and taking notes in the library without depending on anyone.

'Guess what! We have Zubin Petit instead of Maya Mehta, today for the English lecture', said Nicky.

'Who is he?', I asked casually.

'He was a student last year at Xavier's, and he is the Teacher's Pet', said Nargis, 'the teacher being Uma'.

'Oh my god! That's the bell. Let's go to the lift. What are you all doing? Hurry up', said Becky, as she rushed towards us.

'Where is the lecture?', I asked.

'On the mezzanine floor.'

'Oh hell', I said. We were late as usual. The lecture was to take place in a classroom on the third floor. The lift only took us to the second floor.

I thought to myself, 'Why did Xavier's have to put all the lectures on the third floor, when they know I have difficulty in walking.' Xavier's was following a good policy in agreeing to admit disabled students, but facilities for accessibility were appalling. Anyway, it could not be helped, *c'est la vie*! I had no time to think negatively now.

We entered late. Geeta and Carol were holding me under the arm on both sides. The class had already begun. I hate entering late as I distracted the class. Zubin stopped speaking and waited until we sat down. It was highly embarrassing, and I wished he would carry on teaching. We were studying T.S. Eliot's *Murder in the Cathedral*.

I looked at him closely and paid more attention to him than to Eliot. He was not bad looking, in fact he was dashing.

He was tall, thin, wore spectacles, and had a distinguished Parsi accent. Although he seemed a bit nervous as this was his first day of teaching, he was better than Maya. He had a good command of the English language, and was fluent despite his Parsi accent.

After the end of the lecture, he came towards me and offered to help take me down. From that day onwards, we would always meet at the bottom of the stairs, 10 minutes before class was to begin. He would hold my one arm, I would hold the banister with the other hand, and we would go up together. I thought we managed well.

I was bowled over! We managed well and I liked him instantly. We were to become great friends.

Meanwhile, I was still struggling with Uma's class.

Uma gave all our examination papers back to us.

We had all failed. We dismally walked down to the canteen.

'What shall we do?', I kept asking Carol. I was definitely going to fail.

'Why not ask Zubin?', Carol suggested. I was hesitant and embarrassed to ask.

One day Uma had organized a screening of *Hamlet* at the Russian Consulate and insisted that we all should attend it. The gang and Zubin piled in to my car. *Hamlet* was dubbed in Russian but there were English subtitles. I found it highly difficult to follow the movie, as the subtitles were zooming too fast for me to absorb. I turned to Zubin who was sitting next to me, and he narrated the story to me in simple English.

One day after the most intimidating lecture with Uma, I mustered up the courage and went up to Zubin, after exchanging the usual pleasantries, I asked him, 'Can you help me?'

'What with?', he said.

'I can't understand T.S. Eliot. It's all Greek to me', I said in my garbled way.

'Okay', he said, 'Why not?, I'll help you. Where shall we meet?'

'Shall we meet at home?', I said, 'We have more space.'

'Sure.'

I gave him my address. We arranged a date to meet.

Zubin started coming home. My Mother and Zubin clicked immediately as she herself had been a student of English. My understanding of Eliot evolved. I slowly began to fathom his material. Eliot propounded a great deal of philosophy which I enjoyed talking about and discussing with Zubin.

Zubin slowly began to understand my speech. By talking about Eliot, my ideas began to develop. I loved talking to Zubin about Eliot. Slowly, we weaved in my disability into the conversations, and started developing a philosophical discussion in regard to my disability. We had endless discussions on what was really therapy for me. I began to verbalize my pain of being and coping in a normal world. He had a loving tone in which he would tackle all questions about my disability and encourage me to talk about what was bothering me.

I began to love *The Wasteland*! We got to know each other through the poem. As we got more into it, we found that we had a great deal in common and enjoyed each other's company.

Zubin became a part of the family. He used to spend hours talking to mother. Mother gave him a part-time job at the Society. Mother was always on the look out for writers to write about the Society. Zubin loved the work and the people in the organization loved Zubin.

We began being invited to the same parties, and ended up dancing together as he was the only one from the opposite sex who could handle me extremely well. He understood my speech completely. I found him to be warm, compassionate and caring. My affection for him grew deeper and deeper.

I passed the second year and was in my final year of the degree. I dropped English and Psychology. I did six papers in History as I found remembering dates and events slightly easier. By the fifth year, I was a well-known figure at Xavier's.

I left the group who stayed on to read six papers in English.

I met up with two old friends from the eleventh and twelfth, Bhavna and Asha, who wrote my notes meticulously. They were thorough in their note-taking which helped me immensely for when I was revising. We had a history teacher called Augusta Perrier who taught three papers, on Europe, America and Asia. It was a secret joke in the class that Augusta had a penchant for Napoleon.

The other three papers on India began with the Indus Civilization; moved through the various dynasties, like the Guptas, the Cholas and India as it was before the Muslim invasion; a study of the art and architecture and the literature written at that time. We studied the various sects of Hinduism, how Jainism and Buddhism emerged out of Hinduism and the four stages in a man's life according to the Hindu religion. One paper was Mughul India, from the time that Babar won the Battle of Panipat to Aurangzeb's reign.

My mother again tirelessly helped me by taking up my work and writing model answers which I cheerfully and unashamedly mugged.

I had four writers. Zubin was one of them. Miss Madan, Varsha and Mangala were the other writers. They patiently listened while I vocalized each word; the Canon Communicator would always be there, in case they did not understand the odd word. My writers had to understand Ancient Indian Sanskrit words which sounded like tongue twisters, such as *Dasadhama*, *Tirthankaras* and *Anupreksha*.

When the time came for negotiating the choice of writers and the amount of time I was to be given, there were again problems, as people knew little or nothing of my difficulties. People from the Spastics Society had to visit the University each day, teaching and familiarizing the staff about dealing with the differently abled. Without their help, I could not have made it.

The BA exam was torturous. This time each paper was six hours long. It seemed as if it were interminable.

Six hours of continuous regurgitation. The worst thing was that the exam took place in the heat of May, when temperatures soared. My throat got so dry calling out long essay type of answers that I could not speak without sips of water. I called out each word laboriously, sometimes spelling it out. We would have a much needed break for lunch. It needed a great deal of patience from the writer too as they listened to my dysarthric speech. The whole process was an arduous one for both the writer and me. We were both ready to be placed on to stretchers at the end of each exam. This must have been what hard labour was like in one of Hitler's concentration camps.

It was late July. The results were out. The first floor was packed with students who were chattering away.

'Malini you have passed', shrieked Bhavna.

I had not done brilliantly, but I did not care. The important thing was that I had passed.

Was it worth it? I often asked myself.

Those physical barriers, the effort of going up those endless stairs with two people on either side; those piercing eyes, hundreds of which would turn to you to stare; those laborious and endless exams going beyond the threshold of tolerance; was it worth it all?

The agony of trying constantly to be understood; the desire to be perceived as normal; the embarrassment of being excluded?

And the positive moments, the sheer joy of being included in the odd picnic, the lunch party, the cinema and even the blacklisting. Above all, the joy of making it through those terrible exams. Those great and glorious days combined with the pain of self-realization, the difficulty in grappling with reality, the endless questioning of whether the world is with me.

Yes, it was worth it, every time, every moment.

We all congratulated each other and went down to the canteen to have our last cup of *chai* under the tree. As I moved in my wheelchair under the large *peepal* tree in the canteen, I had a sudden desire to cry.

I realized that my first experience in the midst of normal people had been a success. I would rather work it out, confronting the situation, instead of being put away in a special school.

I was Malini Chib, BA!

Introdution to Port Wine
Goa with Nicky

'Why don't you come along to Goa with me?', suggested Nick one day. He was now in the United States, completing a Liberal Arts degree from the University of Rochester (or U of R, as they called it). As is common in America, it was a broad-based degree with many options available—including the option to spend a year studying abroad. He had selected the Institute of Human Potential in Vienna, where he was studying Psychology and Psychiatry. His friend Alison, who was studying at the Institute of European Studies, had come with him to India, for a holiday.

My eyes lit up on hearing his invitation. I hugged him and danced around with delight. To be in Goa would be wonderful, especially with my 22-year-old brother Nick.

'I take that means a yes', said Nick, who always spoke in a sardonic, humorous manner.

'Yes, yes, I'd love to come!' I said, 'but how you will manage the practicalities of both me and the wheelchair all by yourself?' I asked him. 'You know I can manage Buck (I had given my wheelchair a name) better than anyone else', responded my brother. 'Also, Alison will help.' I laughed happily and blew him a kiss.

We left the next morning. Bombay airport knew my needs well. With the help of the kind ladies from the facility counter, we sailed through the airport without difficulty. Goa was only 45 minutes away by air.

It was the beginning of April and the summer was just weeks away. Although the days were hot, it was not sultry or unbearable. There was a constant cool breeze from the Arabian Sea, making it very Mediterranean-like and pleasant.

We arrived at mid-day, only to be accosted by taxi drivers who, realizing we were tourists, were all too eager to make a quick rupee or two. Unlike other parts of India, the locals in Goa, if presented with the opportunity, are quick to take you for a ride, no matter what skin colour you may be. My brother knew the system well and arranged something for us within seconds.

Our destination was Baga Beach, North Goa. The journey to our hotel was picturesque, despite the uneven roads, which made me feel slightly car-sick. The crops were a yellowish dusty colour and were waiting for the monsoons to change back to their natural luscious green. The road had been newly built. When we were children, we would often go to Goa by ferry, crossing the river Mandovi.

My excitement to travel to Goa with Nick had not abated. Although we had grown up together, I was longing to discover the adult Nick. This was the first time Nick was alone with me, without the family. I also loved to be with my own generation, which is a rare occasion for me. I tend to spend more time with my parents' generation.

We got to Baga around 2 pm and went straight to Erica's boutique, as we were staying with her. Erica and her sister Joanne had come to India from South Africa 20 years ago. They were friends of *kaka*. They had completely imbibed the lifestyle of Goa and had made themselves a part of the life in Baga. Both sisters were oversized but looked good in their exotic, loose westernized clothes, which they designed and which showed off their gorgeous tan. Although they were loud and highly eccentric, they were warm.

Alison, who was from Texas, was a typical American tourist. She wanted a quick whirlwind tour of Goa's churches and beaches with Nick alone and did not quite understand the Indian way of family life where sisters are included. She was pleasant enough but she would sulk if things did not go according to her wishes. She would wander off on her own as she was keen on sightseeing, whereas Nick and I had seen the sights of Goa on our previous visits and much preferred to laze around soaking up the sun.

'I hope you don't mind Alison, the loo is Indian style', said Erica, casually. She probably thought that it was only Alison who would be affected, being a foreigner.

My heart fell. I was not used to an Indian style toilet. An Indian style toilet needs quite some skill and manoeuvrability. One has to balance in a squatting position to spend a penny, which is all very well for the rest of humanity who possess good balance, but not an easy task for someone like me, who suffers from ataxia and has limited balance. I had been to Goa many times before but this was the first time I had to experience this style of emptying one's bladder.

'You have used this kind of loo before, haven't you?', asked Erica. I nodded apprehensively. I was dying to talk to Nick so as to sort out the matter, but Erica was chattering with Alison, suggesting places that she should see.

'How are we going to manage?', I thought to myself. Nick, who could see my anxiety, kept telling me in Bengali (our secret language), 'Don't worry, we will discuss it later.'

I was not going to let the excitement of having Nick all to myself be dampened by a stupid method of ablution. We were surprised to discover that in the whole of Baga, there was only one public western-style loo and that too in a small little café on the beach, known as Anthony's. Anthony (the owner) had the key, so we had to go and ask for the key every time I wanted to use it. We had to leave Buck outside, as the loo was small and had just enough space to fit Nick and me. Nick, being a frenetic for hygiene and cleanliness, decided to meticulously put toilet paper around the seat, as he was constantly afraid of catching a disease. He helped me on the seat and stood patiently in the corner until I finished my business. This was a daily ceremony, which he performed diligently.

Nick's concern for me left a lump in my throat.

Oh, it was fabulous to be in Goa. The smell of the sea air greeted us with open arms. It was so soothing and peaceful to be away from the hectic life that I had led in Bombay in the last few months. We shed our city clothes, slipped into our beach-wear and with our books in tow, headed towards Baga Beach. If one was observant, one could see nude hippies sunbathing. The beach looked ravishing. It was a landscape composed of white sand and clear blue water, with rustic boats scattered along Monet style, waiting to be taken out to fish by the locals.

Being of a highly adventurous disposition, Nick was dying to spend a night with the locals and to go fishing with them at sunset. The best fish can only be caught at night. Every time the subject came up, I hoped that he was only kidding. Erica, aware of my trepidation, ensured that we were booked every evening, thank goodness.

We had difficulty in getting the wheelchair down to the sea, as the sand can be a tedious surface to tread on, but Nick managed it beautifully. He was familiar with manoeuvring the wheelchair and he knew how to handle it well on the rickety, uneven paths of Goa. Although Goa was not a very friendly place for my wheelchair, it did not deter us from taking it to the sea.

Our days were relaxed as we spent most of the afternoon basking in the sun. I often thought of my stepmother Margot, who was quite enthusiastic about getting enough sun. Whenever she saw me, she would say, 'Darling, you are so white, you need the sun. Why don't you come with me on Sunday morning to the club?' She would bask in the sun there, wearing a bikini.

In my college days, my beauty sleep was a more important concern. I used to wake up at 7 am on weekdays, so I would routinely decline her kind invitation, not wanting to sacrifice the luxury of waking up late. Margot and I had become very close; she was my good friend. She was obviously nothing like a traditional stepmother. I kept thinking about how lucky I was to have such an exceptional family.

When the sun retired for the day, we went to Anthony's, a beach café that was the favourite amongst Nick and his crowd of friends. Anthony's was a barn type restaurant. We began the evening with a round of drinks and starters consisting of prawns and mussels made in the Goan style. I could not believe that Goan Port Wine was sold for ₹ 9, so you can guess how many glasses I had. It was my first introduction to Port Wine and I loved it.

'You guys are late', cried Erica, one night, in her Anglo-Indian accent, as we strolled in lazily. Our bodies were covered with sand and we were feeling dirty and grimy. 'Please hurry up. My friend Christina is throwing a party for all of you', she said. We just about managed to have a decent wash in the cramped bathroom and off we went to this party which was full of people who were either high on drugs or booze. It was one of those palatial British Raj bungalows with a huge garden. Pockets of people were scattered over the lawns.

I spent half of the evening counselling Alison who, through the course of this trip, had come to see Nick in a new light. She remarked that Nick seemed like a stranger but to me, he was behaving like his usual self. Perhaps he was not paying her enough attention. Nick had changed back to being his old self and was mixing with all sorts of people. Although their relationship was platonic, it was obvious that she liked him. I think Alison was envisaging cosy romantic evenings and candlelit dinners with Nicky on the beaches of Goa. Instead, she found a mass of local people surrounding him and gaping at him as if he was a Greek god. There was also his constant preoccupation with his disabled sister. I tried half heartedly to get to know her, but I soon lost interest.

At the party, I decided to investigate how much Goan Wine I could drink. I knew that it was a worthless endeavour to prove my intelligence that evening and I was happy to just sit and listen to people's chatter. I hadn't felt this relaxed in a long time. My glass was repeatedly refilled by Erica who thought that I was cute because I was on a wheelchair. I laughed a great deal at her jokes. There were people who were affectionate, nurturing and patronizing because I was with Buck. Nick sat in the distance, giving me disapproving glances, which I chose to ignore. I was obviously getting slowly but surely inebriated.

I only managed to drink half the bottle and I was completely drunk. I flopped onto Nick's shoulder in the car. Nick was petrified as he thought I was going to die. My head was spinning and I thought this was the end. Nick helped me with my nightclothes and instructed me to have a glass of water which was a mistake because I promptly vomited all over Nick and Buck. Meticulously, Nicky cleaned up the mess and I vowed never to drink again. But that vow lasted only until sunset the next evening.

I will always remember the beautiful, caring and relaxed holiday with my brother.

Entre-vous to Adulthood

After my degree, I went to the United States for a short visit in 1988. It was a great learning experience for me. One of the places I visited was Berkeley.

When visiting the University town of Berkeley, I was pleasantly surprised to find it teeming with electric wheelchairs; in fact, these wheelchairs were the order of the day. Wheelchairs had the right of way. The traffic came to a halt just to let them cross the road. The accessibility was splendid. All the pavements were ramped and the curbs rounded, making it a very disabled-friendly place. A wheelchair could hop on and off with ease. Every place was accessible, be it a library, museum, restaurant, shop, school, public toilet or theatre, and this facilitated independence. In fact, the campus is located on a hill, and it is advisable for a disabled person to have an electric wheelchair. Besides mobility, it gives a disabled person a sense of freedom, making one forget that he or she cannot walk. It was unbelievable for me, coming from a country where most buildings are totally inaccessible to wheelchairs. Often I have been upset while trying to enter five-star hotels, art galleries, or parks in India, to find that no thought has been given to a person who cannot walk. Usually, all that is needed is a ramp.

In Berkeley, there were several organizations dealing with disabled students and fighting for the rights of disabled people. We visited the Centre for Independent Living. At the centre, they train disabled people on how to manage their lives, even if they suffer from severe disabilities. Disabled people had the help of many different attendants who aided them with daily living functions, keeping in mind their needs. Dad and I saw many disabled adults with multiple attendants who came and went. What I found hugely amazing was that disabled people themselves were in charge and were placed in positions of power. They hired, and fired their personal helpers, who were called attendants. I saw many disabled people like me, or more severe than me, in positions of power, heading disability organizations. In Berkeley, disabled people prefer hiring outsiders and not their own family and friends to assist them, as this brings in a neutral person, and obfuscates some level of emotional attachment.

Disabled people in Berkeley argue that all people are interdependent.

They argue that nobody is completely independent. For instance, a normal person would need a carpenter, a plumber or an electrician, perhaps. The disabled, too, are dependent on getting help to enable independent living, so that they can function more efficiently and are able to take up employment. Therefore, a personal attendant is really one's hands and legs in the form of another human being. The disabled person instructs his attendant about the ways and means he would like to be helped. He is taught how to train his or her own personal attendant, to hire as well as to fire. To me, this form of independence is essential if I am to be allowed to contribute positively to society, and not always be treated as a second-class citizen because I need help with my personal care. Again this kind of philosophy was new to me.

This concept appealed to me a great deal. Society always has these stereotypical concepts of disabled people, where they are portrayed as being extremely dependent and helpless. Why? Disabled people are human beings first. But most people see the deformity and the disability before they notice any personal attributes. The person within the disabled person is always unnoticed because their physical demands are so immense and often glaring. I am sure most disabled people think so. The disabled person requires so much help that often the career gets burnt out. Over the years, I have learnt that a disabled person must depend on many people for him/her to lead a so-called normal life.

It was after my trip to Berkeley that we decided to get an attendant. Mother was in Calcutta at the time. She interviewed a Nepalese woman who spoke English. Maya was pleasant, and in her mid-forties. Her last employers were one of the elite families of Calcutta.

Maya arrived a month later. She had a pleasant disposition. Actually she was a great help to my mother and Pam. For the first time in years, we had a maid for our clothes.

Maya came and helped me with my daily living needs. In Berkeley, disabled people called an aide a personal attendant. I was 22 and could no longer be dependent on mother for my physical care.

Maya was a new addition to my new life. My trip to the US was an eye-opener for me. I had never seen so many disabled adults in my life, each leading an independent life. In Bombay when I was growing up, I rarely saw a disabled adult. So I invariably grew up thinking that I would be normal once I was an adult.

My mother would always ask, 'When are you going be independent?'

'When I grow up', I would say.

'And that is when? Please tell me', said mother. 'You are already 21.'

Today, when I reflect on the past, I realize that my growing up started when I left home and went to Oxford. It was after our trip to Berkeley, when we had stopped over in London prior to returning to Bombay, that one day, dad asked casually, 'Molls, shall we go to Oxford Polytechnic?' He rang up Oxford Polytechnic and spoke to the Dean who gave us a time to meet with him. We hired a Hertz and drove down to Oxford, which was an hour's drive.

The Polytechnics of Britain offer a technical training, which the universities did not offer. It was only recently that the Polytechnics were formally recognized as universities. I felt that I needed a more practical training to get a job. With my poor speech, I thought that formal training would give me an edge over others. Oxford Polytechnic had a good course in Publishing. I decided to apply with dad's help. I put in the application and was called for the interview.

The interview was most informal. The Dean wore a white checked crumpled shirt. It was like an informal chat.

When I returned to Bombay, I did not give it a single thought. I immersed myself in the work of the Spastics Society. I decided to set up an informal recreational club called ADAPT (Able Disabled All People Together), where people could meet socially, as I felt that there was not much interaction between non-disabled and disabled people. My friend, Zubin, and I thought up the name ADAPT at the same time, which was coincidental. ADAPT met every two weeks just as a social forum.

Zubin and I spent hours together, talking and getting to know each other.

'I would like to go to England to study Chaucer', said Zubin.

'Why don't you apply to Oxford and try for a scholarship?'

'It's not easy Molls.'

'Come on, why don't you apply and give it a shot?', I said.

'Okay, I will think about it', said Zubin.

He applied and got an interview. *Mesho* (my uncle) was on the board of the Inlaks Scholarship. However, Zubin was indeed a brilliant scholar and certainly did not need anyone to pull any strings for him.

'Molls I got it!' Zubin exclaimed as he gave me a hug.

'Congrats', I said. It was a mixture of joy and sadness. My best friend would be leaving Bombay and yet I felt happy that he had got into Oxford.

Zubin left for Oxford.

I felt sad at seeing him go. I buried myself in the work of the research department of the Spastics Society.

One morning out of the blue, a letter arrived. The heading on the envelope was marked 'Oxford Polytechnic'.

Mother opened the letter. The letter said:

Dear Ms Chib,
I hereby inform you that you have been accepted in the publishing course.

On reading the letter, I shrieked with joy.

Mother hugged me and said, 'You must get a scholarship otherwise you will not be able to go.'

Mother always tried to make me see the reality. I crossed my fingers, hoping to get the money. I was slowly entering adulthood.

I counted the days when I would be in Oxford. I was not sure whether I was looking forward to being at Oxford or being with Zubin.

Oxford: A Love Affair

Oxford is famous for its beauty, atmosphere and, of course, the knowledge and learning it imparts. It is unlike any other city in the world. Its uniqueness lies in its mellow beauty and architectural elegance, crowned by the glory of the ancient colleges. The ambience of Oxford, I decided, was infectious for students. You get hooked on to the city. With a family legacy comprising of an education in the Oxbridge tradition, I was keen to spend some time there, and I was pleased when I got admitted into the Oxford Polytechnic, which is now known as Brookes University. I might not have been in one of the famous ancient colleges, but I was in OXFORD.

As soon as I arrived in Oxford, I met with Zubin. It was lovely to see him and I felt instantly comfortable as he greeted me with special warmth and affection. My initiation to Oxford began with Zubin and I taking long walks, with him serving as a tour guide of sorts, showing me around. Zubin told me about the Town and Gown concept. The Town and Gown are two distinct communities of the university town, where 'Town' refers to the non-academic population and 'Gown' refers to the university community, especially, the ancient seats of learning that were in essence what Oxford and Cambridge stood for.

'I will take you to the University of Oxford Botanic Garden', said Zubin one day.

The Oxford Botanic Garden is a scientific garden. It is one of the oldest botanic gardens in the world and the oldest in Great Britain. The garden was established in 1621 and contains specialist plant collections, with many plants suited to medical research. It is a lush space full of greenery and spread out over 4 acres, situated in the city centre.

I loved the botanic garden.

We walked through the walled garden admiring the 17th century stonework, stopping to look at the garden's oldest tree, an English Yew. The garden was dotted with glasshouses, the presence of which makes possible the cultivation of plants not naturally suited to England's harsh and extreme weather conditions.

I could see a lot of tropical plants like the ones we see in India. The British have carefully brought and grown them here.

'Molls, the collection of plants which are grown here, are not only for aesthetic reasons. Many gardeners come here to seek inspiration. In the beds and borders you may discover new species of plants that would be perfect in your garden at home, and partly for this reason, they strive to clearly label every plant in the garden', said Zubin as we walked around the ravishing gardens.

Zubin was always perfectly comfortable with me. It is because he understood my speech completely and was one of those few human beings who did not need another person to escort me when we spent time together. He could wheel me around everywhere. Some people preferred the assistance of an interpreter or someone to manage the wheelchair, but Zubin managed me and the wheelchair entirely on his own.

Secretly, I always hoped for a relationship wherein Zubin and I could be more than just friends. He was kind, loving, patient and always there for his friends.

About a month or two before I was to arrive in Oxford, Dad, with Zubin's help, had found a flat for me. It was a quaint, lovely, semi-detached, two bedroom flat, near the famous Oxford Shark. The Headington Shark, as it is called, is a sculpture depicting a shark embedded head-first in the roof of a residential house. It was created by an architect called John Buckley, who owns this unique house adorned with a shark emerging through the roof. The Shark was a controversial issue when it first appeared, as the residents of Headington wanted it to be pulled down. But later Buckley received an award and the shark has quickly become a tourist favourite.

However, mother was not too happy to leave me with the carer in this area.

'It is too isolating for Malini and Maya', said mother to dad. 'Let's look for something else.' Dad went to see if he could find student accommodation where both Maya and I could live. Luckily, he found a student residence called Pollock House advertised on the Oxford Brookes Bulletin Board. 'You are lucky Sir, we have one disability friendly room', said Helen Green, the Accommodation Officer.

'How wonderful! When could we have a look?', asked dad.

'I can show you at 6 pm', said Helen.

'Fine. I will bring Molls', said dad.

We saw the house. It was a huge Victorian Mansion. Pollock House is located in Pullens Lane in Headington, and is very close to Oxford Polytechnic. It is located at the top of Headington Hill.

Originally named 'the Vineyard', the house was renamed 'Pollock House' once it was acquired by the United Oxford Hospitals in 1948. For a few years it served as a Nurse's training school after which it was converted into a Night Nurses' Home. In 1976, Oxford Polytechnic bought the property and made it into a Student's Hostel, by renovating it into 10–12 student rooms.

Maya and I were assigned a huge, spacious room overlooking a beautiful, massive garden. There was ample space for two beds and both Maya and I had our privacy. There was a shared adapted toilet for disabled people at the end of the corridor. There was a common kitchen for all students, which became the hub of gossip and exchange in the evening when we cooked dinner together, sharing our food with each other.

The view from my room was breathtaking. When we drew the curtains we could see a gigantic garden, which with its luscious green landscape, was an exquisite feast for the eyes. The grounds of the garden were shared by the students of Oxford Polytechnic and Robert Maxwell, the well known Media Baron. Of course, his side of the property was huge and beautifully laid out.

The students were mature and friendly. Fortunately for me, Maya was fluent in English which was very useful considering my impaired speech.

Maya was extremely fond of certain soaps that were aired on TV.

'I must watch "Neighbours"', Maya said one evening. 'I want to know what is happening to Kylie.' Due to her knowledge of English, Maya fit into student life at Pollock House well. Students would love to have a quick cup of tea with her, and soon she was the star of Pollock House, immensely liked by all.

We were never lonely in Pollock House. Maya, like me, had the great ability to make friends. We were frequently invited out. There would always be someone around to have a chat with. It is important when a carer and a disabled person live together that both of them have outlets of their own, otherwise the relationship can become strenuous and suffocating.

Ever since I threw myself into the world of normal people, first at Xavier's and then at Oxford, I have not stopped thinking about my added disability of poor speech. Having had carers not as proficient in English as Maya, I have realized one thing for certain—when a person with disability has the added handicap of poor speech, it is necessary for the attendant or friend with her to speak fluent English, especially if one is in England. However, being with Maya had its set of advantages and disadvantages. The problem with having a carer who is fluent, as Maya was, is that it was easier for people to ignore me and address the carer instead. Most people are afraid of not understanding me, because they are afraid of the unknown. When accompanied by a carer, there is always the danger of being overlooked and passed over by the carer's propensity to make casual conversation. Trained carers do not allow themselves to take over. Maya was lovely. She never took over and was very careful to include me. We had a vast circle of friends.

An old childhood friend called Navina was in Oxford. Navina had the gift of recounting stories in a humorous way. I marveled at her ability to transform painful elements of a story into an amusing account.

There were two couples who were particularly friendly towards us, namely, Jabir and Rukshana from Bangladesh, and Sue and Graham. They were always there to keep an eye on us, and provide any assistance if needed. There were other students like me who also had special needs. Peter was Hemophilic, Graham had become disabled after a car-accident, and Damien was on a wheelchair. Graham had been sent to University by his office. He said that he derived his strength from me as I was an inspiration. We had long talks about being disabled. During our conversations, I often realized that when it came to our attitude towards life, I seemed to be the stronger one. Perhaps I had been shielded from the harsh realities of life until now.

Maya and I immediately warmed up to Jabir and Rukhsana. Maya had an advantage in that, being from Darjeeling, she spoke fluent Bengali.

'Today you will eat with us because we have brought fresh *Ilish* (Hilsa) fish from Cowley Road', said Jabir. Ilish is the queen of Bengali fish and extremely popular in Bengali cuisine.

'We would love to come', I said, as I had often had it at home and at my grandmother's place. Sue and Graham were also invited. The conversation at the dinner table was pleasant and full of revelry. Graham related his plans to solve the world's problems. Sue reminded me of Pam. She was really a lot of fun.

'Hi', said Sue.

'Hi, I love your skirt and jumper', I said.

'I brought it at the car boot sale for £2.'

'How affordable! Maya and I would love to go there', I said.

So the next weekend, Maya and I piled into their car. The car boot sale was a nifty idea. People brought their old unwanted clothes and knick-knacks which they did not use and sold it at a low price. For students, the car boot sale was an excellent find. My wardrobe expanded twice a month, as I picked up trendy yet affordable items.

It was a cold winter day when the bell at Pullock House rang. I hoped that other inmates of the house would answer it. No such luck. I went on my wheelchair and was delighted to see Uncle Yogesh and his son Vickram.

That evening, Navina, Vickram and I went out together. 'What do you want to do after you finish your degree in Oxford?', Navina asked Vickram. Navina and I had become great friends as our parents knew each other. We were sitting in the courtyard of one of the famous pubs which had tall weeping willow trees.

'Navina, I want to go into all the villages of India and educate the masses', said Vickram.

'How are you going to do that?', we asked.

'Well, I am thinking of a plan, once I have one I will let you know', he said.

'Please let us know when you start it, we would love to help', I said.

'Your ideas are so obscure. I do hope they become a reality, then you can win a Padmashri', joked Navina.

Such conversations, filled with big dreams and ambitious plans in a lighthearted setting, is what I loved about my life in Oxford.

I readily settled into life at Oxford, learning to balance my classes and my social life.

My Publishing Course was for a year. It was meant for professionals who were keen on working in the industry. The course taught us all aspects of publishing, including editorial processes, design and layout, copywriting material, using computer software, the financial aspects of publication, the intricacies of the production process and marketing.

Again, like there had been at Xavier's, there were access problems. The Publishing Department was up one flight of stairs, so when I wanted to meet my tutors, I had to walk up with Maya and always prearrange these visits as the effort was only worth it if I was guaranteed a meeting. It was physically fatiguing and prevented me from using the Department's facilities.

I had two tutors, Kevlin Smith and Bob Woodings. Initially, they were both a bit apprehensive about how I would finish the course. My incomprehensible speech made them doubt my intelligence.

Zubin and Navina were readily available for assistance during tutorials to help interpret my speech.

I had a lot to learn because I had little exposure to the publishing world. There were 20 of us in class. My classmates were all working in different parts of the world and for many I was the first disabled person they had met.

Looking back, my interaction with my classmates was more like integration, as although the students were friendly, I felt that they could have been more helpful. I had to repeatedly ask them for notes, which they were finicky about sharing; they much preferred to keep their notes to themselves. I missed my friends at Xavier's who were helpful and inclusive and would always lend me their notes. Again, I had difficulties with accessing the library. The library was a bit of a trek away and getting to it was a physically demanding task. The Polytechnic library had a disabled entrance but disabled students had to alert the librarian when they were planning to come. Also, there was no orientation to familiarize us with the use of the library.

Dad and Zubin often helped me with my assignments as my written work was not technical enough. This can partly be attributed to the fact that I had attended a special school for eight years, as I earlier have explained, because of which my writing was affected. I think one of the fundamental concerns for education for disabled people is the communication output. Special and inclusive educators should first look at the child's communication needs as the primary concern. I managed to get by with their help.

The last and final model of the course was Desktop Publishing. We had to publish two books. I did Zubin's book, which was a book of poems titled *Small Moves* and I put together one of my mother's short paper entitled 'The History of Special Education in India'.

As part of the course, all students were to have a mock interview for a job in a publishing house and this was to count towards 30 per cent of the grade. I was looking forward to it, as I had never experienced a viva before. But as the days progressed, I heard rumours from others in the class that the two professors were very tough.

'Malini, everybody has to have a viva. How will you do it? We have to find a way', said Kevlin.

'I will get an interpreter', I said quickly. When one is disabled, one has to make it easier for themselves in the normal world. You cannot expect the world to do everything for you.

The days passed by quickly. Before I knew it, the day for my interview had arrived. I was nervous as I was convinced that I did not know very much. I took Zubin along as my interpreter. The interview was tough as Kevlin and Bob grilled me. Question after question was fired at me. I had to speak articulately.

There was no beating around the bush. Every ounce of knowledge I had, I regurgitated. Forty-five minutes later Kevlin told me that I had got the job.

I smiled.

'I wish it was for real', I joked.

I did well and passed. I had come a full circle in one year. A year ago, my professors knew nothing about me as a student with special needs, but after dealing with me for the year, they no longer thought my problems were insurmountable.

So, yes, there was good news, I was doing well in class, making new friends and enjoying my time with old ones, Zubin especially. What happened next was something I least expected.

'Molls, I have to talk to you about something', Zubin said one evening. He sounded very solemn. We were taking one of our routine walks in the botanic garden.

'What is it?', I said anxiously.

'Molls, I am gay', he said

I could not quite understand.

'I love men sexually', Zubin explained, 'I have a partner from Belgium and his name is Bart. He is coming here in a few weeks and you must meet him. I know you both will like each other immensely.'

I did not show my emotions right away. Perhaps, I did not yet fully realize how badly this was going to impact me. When Zubin left me, I started crying. Why was I crying?

Yes, I was deeply hurt. For days, I would go off on my own and have a silent weep. I must have silently desired a more romantic relationship. I was 21 and wanted male attention. All my girlfriends had boyfriends and, I too, wanted a boyfriend. Why could not I be in a relationship? What was so abnormal about me? I could not comprehend my emotions. I yearned for all that was normal despite my disabled body.

What made things worse was that Zubin understood me perfectly. We had shared a great deal together and had so much in common. I heard later from a common friend, Helen, that Zubin was also upset and had admitted that if had he not been gay, he would have been with me.

For me it was a devastating heartbreak. It was not to be. The realization saddened me.

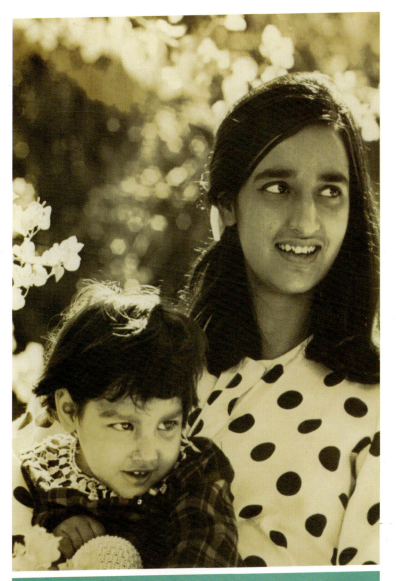
Mother and me when we returned back to India

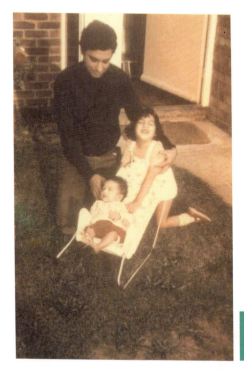

Nikhil (baby), Kaka and me in the garden outside our home in Richmond, England

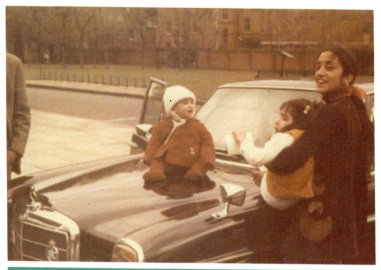

My aunt Juniema with Nikhil (on the car bonnet) and me in London

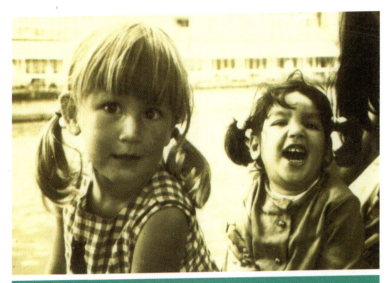

An East-West friendship with Fiona Banes, both aged 2!

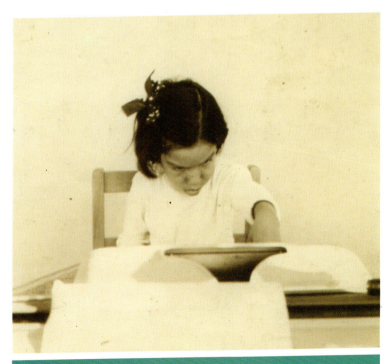

One little finger begins to work. Me, aged 6, with the typewriter

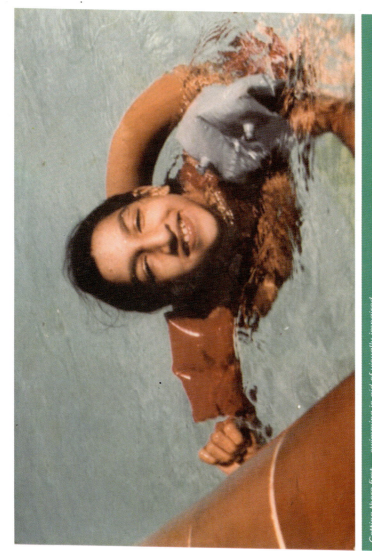

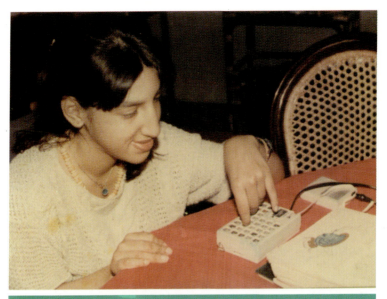

My one little finger working at age 16 …

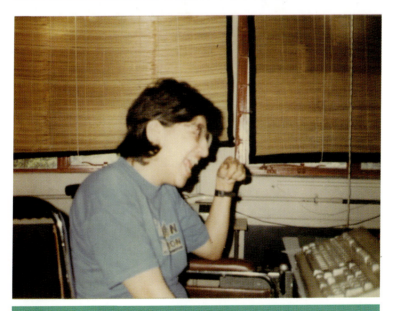

One little finger continues at age 25 … now on a computer!

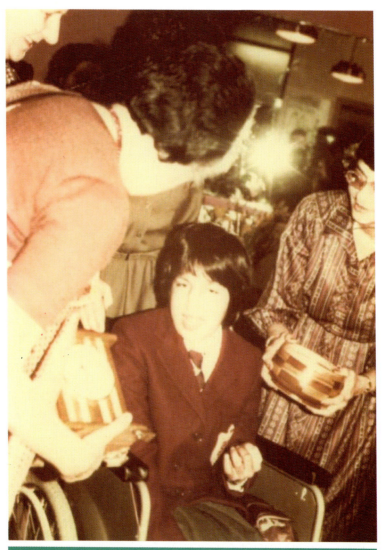

The late Mrs Indira Gandhi opens an SSI exhibition known as 'Action India' at the Spastics Society, UK, and I present her with a clock I put together (1982)

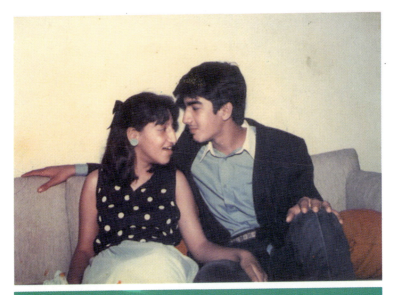

My brother, Nikhil, and me

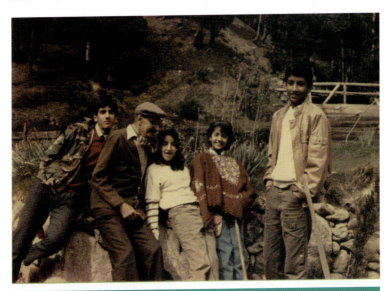

Holiday in Kashmir with barra dada (grandad), and from L to R—Nikhil, me, Karuna and Surajit

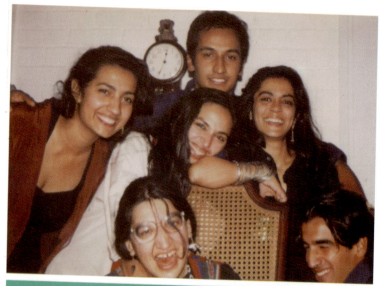

My brothers and sisters

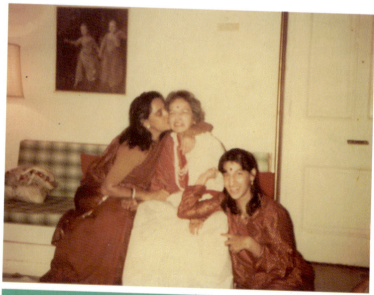

Three generations: Mother (L), ammi (grandmother) and me (R)

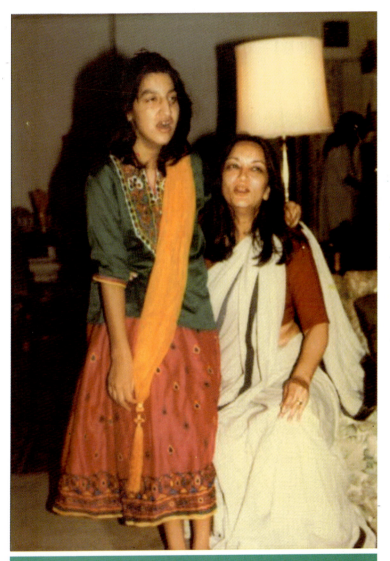
My aunt, Radha, and 21-year-old me at home in Bombay

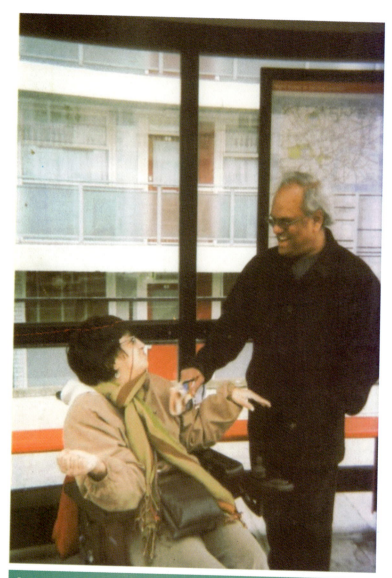
Sathi and me at the London flat (2005)

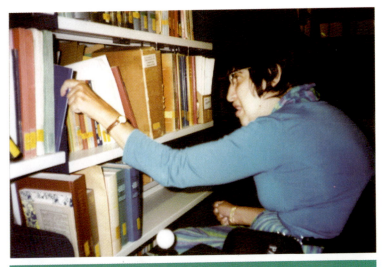

My Masters' Programme at the Institute of Education, London (2002)

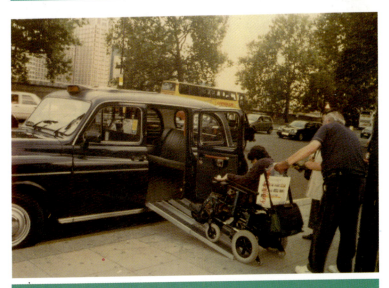

Negotiating the London taxis (2005)

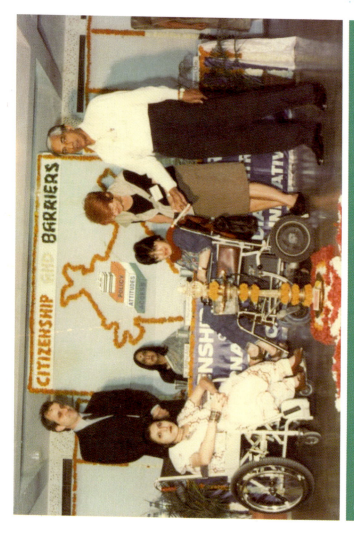

Beginning ADAPT with Citizenship and Barriers Conference, from L to R—Neenu Kelwani, Michael Bach, Dr Mithu Alur, Me, Prof Diana Leonard and then Chief Secretary, Ranganathan, lighting the lamp

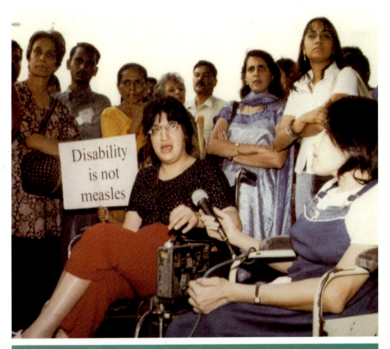

A demonstration by ADAPT (2001)

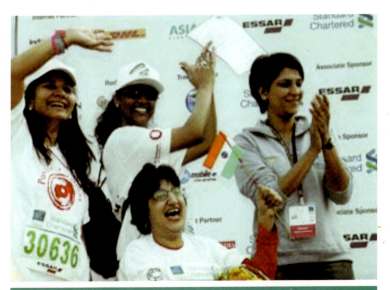

My friends, Priya Dutt (R) and Sunita Rao (C), at the Marathon cheering me

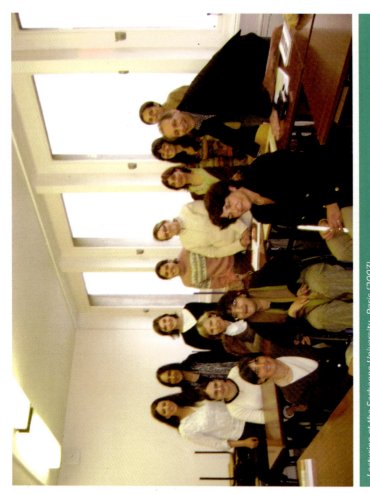

Lecturing at the Sorbonne University, Paris (2007)

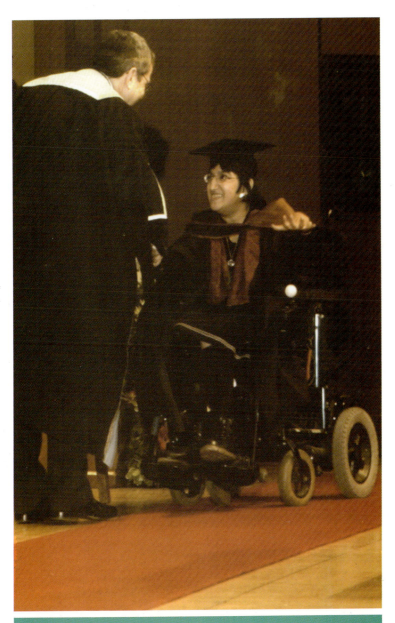

Completing my Masters' in Women's Studies

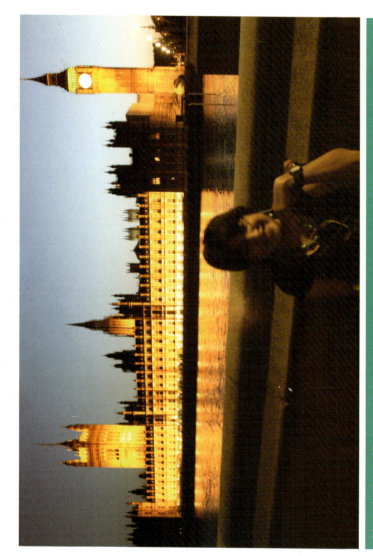

Me, at the House of Parliament, London

Three

A SLICE OF FREEDOM

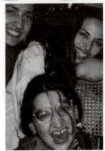

Moving Again to London

Yes, it was hard and lonely to get on with life despite that huge knock. Perhaps life is meant to test you, throwing in your way hard emotional knocks and you just need to spring back like a rubber ball. How else can one cope? My experience is that most people cannot deal with other people's trauma. One's trauma is one's own and should not be mentioned unnecessarily to others. I am reminded of that song by Peter Gabriel, which runs: *Don't Give Up*. I believe in that.

Having completed my one-year course, I was sad to leave Oxford and my idyllic life in Pollock House.

On my return to Bombay, I felt that there was a need for disabled people to socially interact with the so called 'normal' people. I believe that though we all have our own problems, we must make an effort to succeed with our fellow human beings. Perhaps, disabled people have to make more of an effort, who knows? I believe that nobody is perfect; we are all, in some way or the other, disabled. Our disability is more visible; others have what I like to call, an 'invisible disability'.

I went back to the recreational club that Zubin and I had started and began working diligently. I got a job in Bombay's *Times* for a short period. The attitude of the editor and my colleagues was great, but they did not think about accessibility concerns, which was unfortunate. The canteen was out of reach, so I could never join my colleagues for a cup of coffee or lunch. I felt hugely isolated during lunch time and hated it. I sat on my own in a large vacant space on my desk and ate alone, sticking out like a sore thumb. The basic problem of working in India was the lack of accessibility. Even toilets for people with disabilities were not accessible. As basic a need as that had not been thought out by the authorities. The toilet had one or two steps. Once I fell and was badly hurt. My attendant was with me, but there were no bars, so I fell. I had to leave the job. I missed the social chitter-chatter, but there was no option. I was not able to go out on my own. The pavements are not rounded to be disability friendly. There are too many people and the streets have too many potholes. I was very accepting. But then I did not know anything better. I did not question much.

At Oxford, studying Desk Top Publishing (DTP) had helped me learn PageMaker, Ventura. I became involved in designing leaflets and information booklets for the Spastics Society for the inauguration of their new building in Bandra. The funds had come from Sweden. Kamal Bakshi was the Vice-Chairman of ADAPT and was the then Ambassador of Sweden. Uncle Kamal and Umi aunty, his wife, as I called them, are very close to us. They helped in the development and growth of the Spastics Society, now called ADAPT. Uncle Kamal, our Patron Sunil Dutt and dad raised money from the Church of Sweden. Margaretha Ringstrom, the Director of the Church of Sweden became a great friend of mother's and became involved in our project to build the spectacular and magnificent building in Bandra, which now houses the offices of our society.

Just as I was settling into life in Bombay, meeting up with old friends and busying myself with the Spastics Society, a letter, enclosed in a 'London School of Economics' (LSE) envelope, arrived. It was for mother. I wondered what it was. Mother opened it. She looked quite pleased and handed it to dad who said, 'Darling, of course you must accept it'. Mother had been invited by the LSE to serve in the capacity of an Academic Visitor for a year.

What an honour we all thought.

'Molls, you must come with me of course. What a wonderful experience it will be.' I was in between jobs. I was finding it difficult to sustain a job simply because of accessibility and attitudinal barriers.

'Yes', I beamed excitedly on hearing my mother's invite. I was going to go back to my favourite place and country. It felt like my home, as I had been so easily accepted. There was no problem of toilets and even the buses had ramps. I was sure that the job prospects would be far better for people with disability as well. I would be exposed to more assistive technology and aids. Yes, I was looking forward to going back.

We left Bombay in the middle of September. Mother, Maya and I waved goodbye to our family in Bombay. It was an emotional farewell.

When we arrived in London, we did not have a place to stay. Margaret Yekutiel, a very close friend of mother, was the first person to stay at the Bandra Centre of the Spastic Society when only the scaffolding was up, when she came to Bombay. She knew how difficult it was to find a house in Central London. She requested her sister, Liz, for help and they, Liz and David Nussbaum, immediately opened their own home for us. I do not know of anybody who would have made such a gesture.

Liz and David had a beautiful home in Putney. It was a warm, comfortable space, and had lots of books and a piano. There was a huge garden that one could bury oneself in, and read a book in quiet solitude. For me, greenery was like heaven. I craved for it in Bombay.

Mother and dad were hunting for a flat like maniacs.

'Have we got the *Evening Standard* today?', asked mother as we zoomed past Hyde Park Corner onto Marble Arch. The two main sources with property rental listings were, the *Evening Standard* and the London School of Economics Housing list.

'No, the *Evening Standard* comes out at noon so we will pick it up now', said dad as he drove along the busiest streets of London. He was very good at directions and could drive around with ease in any of the European cities.

'Why don't we look at the LSE listings?', gestured dad, as he handed mother the papers.

'There's one on Baker Street', said mother.

'Molls just see the number. Please call it out', said mother to me as we sat and sipped cold coffee at a Starbucks on Bakers Street. The number had been written in fine print and I could read it despite wearing thick glasses.

'Don't be passive and lazy', said mother. Mother was always urging me to do more to participate.

I called out the number to mother and an appointment was made for 5 o'clock in the evening.

They came back beaming after meeting the landlady of the flat. 'We like it, but it's a bit steep.'

It was a huge three bedroom house with two bathrooms, a spacious kitchen and a central dining room. I had a cosy single room. I used to love reading late, often staying up till the early hours of the morning. We converted the third bedroom into a study. The flat had a massive kitchen where we ate breakfast. The kitchen was a place of solace for Maya, where she loved reading her Nepalese romances. Our friend Bobbie had given me her old Amstrad. It was a simple word processor. I bashed away, attempting short stories and wrote long letters home to the rest of the family in India. At the Baker Street flat, dad loved shopping and bought everything in bulk. Mother had a passion for cooking and the British palette seemed to be fond of her dishes. So we did a lot of entertaining. We stayed in Baker Street for a year. It was a year of luxurious splendour. After a year we had to move. Dad found another, smaller flat on Devonshire Street. Again it was very centrally located; Oxford Street was a stone's throw away. Sometimes, Maya and I would venture into the interior parts of Soho, where Chinatown is, and we used to guzzle down dumplings and Chinese buns. Maya became a good friend. Regent's Park was just round the corner. At this time, *ammi* (my grandmother) came and stayed with us and the three of us would spend a lot of time together in the parks. We would make routine visits to Trafalgar Square and the city's various Museums.

I met up with my friends Rosie and John. Rosie had become a Chaplain of a women's prison in Suffolk. She asked me to talk to the prisoners. What a great experience. Initially they did not know how to react to me. After my talk there were a lot of questions. Looking back, it was definitely one of my best talks.

Most of the time was spent in libraries because of the demands of the PhD. Mother had a very good supervisor, Jennifer Evans, who became a close friend of ours. Through our studies, we found that the old medical model of disability had changed to a rights based approach, which was known as the social model. According to this, if a disabled person could not access to offices, restaurants, libraries et cetera, it was not because she or he could not walk, but because of the faulty design of the environment, or the faulty attitude of society. The old belief that a disabled person had to be fixed, fitted and cured had changed to a more social approach. This definition, made a clear distinction between the impairment itself (such as, a medical condition that makes a person unable to walk) and the disabling effects of society in relation to that impairment. In simple terms, it is not the inability to walk that prevents a person from entering a building unaided, but rather the design or location of stairs that are inaccessible to a wheelchair-user. In other words, 'disability' is socially constructed. Mother read about the critiques against institutionalization, against special schools, entrenched negative policies and shared all this new knowledge each day with me and dad. The current belief was that disabled children should study with their normal peers and this was known as inclusive education. Being educated with their normal peers from a young age meant disabled children were in the mainstream and therefore found it easier to be included in all spheres of life. Today, the social model has taken centre stage which says it is the entrenched exclusionary laws, society's attitudes, the environment and not the person that needs fixing. It was also around that time that the disability movement was born. The slogan for the day was, *nothing for the disabled without disabled people.*

All this fascinated her. It was on her exposure to such ideas, that mother felt the need to study further and do her PhD. Her research was to investigate a particular Government of India policy, known as the Integrated Child Development Scheme (ICDS), the world's largest pre-school policy run by the Government. The ICDS operates amongst the poorest sections of the population in India, for pre-school children in the age range of 0–6 years. Although the ICDS policy states that it is for 'all' children, in practice, it does not address the question of disabled children. The research question was, 'What was the explanation for ICDS not explicitly excluding, but not directly addressing, the needs of the pre-school disabled child within their existing provisions for the weaker and more vulnerable sections of society?' Mother was accepted. The Institute of Education in the University of London was beautifully situated in Bloomsbury. Mother was given a two-room flat on the first floor, usually given to PhD researchers. Bloomsbury could not have been more ideal. Camden, Soho, Leicester Square, the parks, Russell Square, the British Museum—the most happening parts of London were all walking or wheelchair distance for me. Woburn Square was not as plush as Baker Street or Devonshire Street, but it was wonderful. Woburn Square is the smallest of the Bloomsbury Squares and owned by the University of London. Woburn Square was designed by Thomas Cubit and built between 1829 and 1847. It was named after Woburn Abbey, the main country seat of the Duke of Bedford, who developed much of Bloomsbury. The Square was always kept locked and only the residents of the square had access to it (like all squares). The area was very pretty and most of all it was familiar territory for us.

'The only snag in the place is that it is up one flight of stairs', said dad, 'but the location is fantastic.'

The flat was a one bedroom and one living room space. It had a tiny kitchenette and a bathroom; it was small but cosy. In both the rooms there were beautiful large French windows which overlooked the Square. When we woke up and sipped our morning tea, we could hear the peaceful whistling of the plane trees which soothed our spirits and prepared us for the rest of the day.

At the same time Professor Klaus Wedell, who was Director of Special Needs at the Institute of Education and a friend of mothers', invited me and mother to a Communication seminar workshop. We went and heard very articulate disabled people talk about the concept of rights and entitlements. There were people who were more severely disabled than me but all could communicate independently. I seemed hopelessly dependent and helpless compared to them. My speech was incoherent and terribly difficult to understand. It continued to depress me immensely, ever since I was confronted with well-articulated youngsters who would chatter away, albeit nonsense. Often, I would come home from college and would collapse in a pile of tears. To me, communication is like water, the essence of life. What could I do without fluent speech?

Hearing the speakers, we felt that it was important now to be able to communicate independently without needing a third party.

We went to Roehampton Hospital in Putney, for an assessment of my communication difficulties. Initially, I was against the idea of having a big communication device like the one Professor Stephen Hawking has, as it was extremely visible and it made my disability look prominent, but I was recommended a smaller and more compact version called 'The Toby Churchill'. What I liked most was that I could carry it in my handbag. Unfortunately that version only has a male voice with a thick American accent. (I am told that a new version is now available with a female voice.)

With the communicator, it was wonderful at communal gatherings like lectures and parties. I should not leave out my favourite place—the pubs. For the first time I did not need a third party to interpret me. My family and friends seemed to be interested in what I had to say. This empowered me a great deal. I had to be cerebral in my topics of conversation. I had to be up-to-date with the news, reading the *Guardian* and listening to *Radio 4*. It took me ages to remember key points of the current headlines.

I was always ecstatic with the electric wheelchair. The electric wheelchair gave me a tremendous feeling of movement and space. With this, I did not feel as if I could not walk. I did not feel helpless. I could slip into shops, chemists, bookshops, restaurants et cetera. Whatever the so called normal person does, I could do. I did this with ease and it did wonders for my self-confidence. I was whizzing around, with mother and Maya sauntering way behind. Maya had supreme confidence in my sense of direction and always followed me blindly.

When I was with dad, he always walked ahead while I wheeled behind. I realized that I was confident and persevering enough to manage the busiest London roads on my own. I realized that I could go anywhere. In my own mind I was ready to tackle the London streets on my own. Friends used to marvel at how I navigated my wheelchair through hordes of tourists through Leicester Square and Soho without touching anyone. Yes, I had to be careful as I knew how very painful it would be if the wheelchair hit one's leg.

We could not have done anything like this in India. I read somewhere that there were over 1,000 potholes and very little pavement space. The pavements were not rounded, and hence not accessible to wheelchairs. Moving around outdoors is not an easy task in India.

I remember clearly when I actually began negotiating the London streets on my own. I would go out frequently, but was always accompanied by my parents or Maya.

'Can I come and pick you up mum?', I asked one morning. I had just woken up and was still snuggled into my cosy IKEA duvet cover. She was going to the Institute of Education's library to read. It was a beautiful sunny day in London.

'Okay, why don't you come with Maya?', said mother as she took her time in picking out her clothes. Mother took no time to adjust to life in England, and had effortlessly switched to wearing trousers and skirts rather than the usual Indian dress. Mother was always pristinely dressed.

'No, I would rather come on my own', I pleaded. I went on nagging her about how I desired solitude at times. At the age of 28, it was too stifling to be accompanied by someone constantly, I wanted a bit of freedom, to be on my own for a while. 'I will be very careful.' I promised.

Mother reluctantly gave in. 'Okay', she said, adding, 'you always get what you want'. I grinned silently knowing very well that when I want something, I will go out of my way for it.

'Please tell Maya', I said firmly, 'or else she won't listen'.

Maya was petrified. 'Madam, it's dangerous, how can you let her? No Madam, it's too dangerous. I will go with her', she repeatedly said.

'No, we must allow this as it is important to enable Malini to be as independent as possible. What I am learning in my studies is to ensure that disabled people have freedom. Be it the freedom to walk around, or to speak and express. We must encourage them to carry out their day to day activities solely by themselves, which will strengthen them', said mother as she put on her black shoes. 'Let her come on her own, Maya', said mother.

I was very excited, but I did not show it in case Maya changed her mind and decided to come along, which would ruin everything. This was my chance to prove to the world that I could master the London roads without getting hit. It was April and spring was unfolding. The days grew longer as we approached the solstice and the temperature grew warmer. We walked along to Budgens (a supermarket) making inconsequential chatter. Then the moment came when Maya and I had to part ways. She was petrified.

'Okay, bye', I said confidently as I waved goodbye. I must admit that I was a trifle nervous myself, but whizzed along through Gower Street; I passed through University Street onto Woburn Square and onto the concourse of the Institute of Education. I wanted to shriek with joy but restrained myself as I did not want people to assume that I was straight out of space or belonged to a lunatic asylum.

'Oh, hi', said mother as she put her books on the back of my wheelchair. 'Where's Maya?', she asked as though nothing unordinary had happened. 'Don't you remember our conversation in the morning?', I said quietly.

'Oh yes, I'd forgotten. You made it alone. Congratulations darling', said mother. We sauntered home together.

From then on, I went everywhere on my own—to bookshops, supermarkets, parks. I changed several buses to meet friends. For the first time, I could shop on my own. I particularly enjoyed window-shopping and would often go have a look around various supermarkets, clothes shops, sales et cetera. That moment was joyous as I moved onto the track of becoming an empowered disabled adult in London. I remember going in to Dillons, the university Bookshop, once without my light-writer. I wanted a particular book called *Mustn't Grumble* by Lois Keith. For a few moments, I did not know what to do. Then I saw a terminal, which became my saviour. I frantically gestured that I wanted to use the computer. The shopkeeper waited patiently, while I laboriously spelt out the name of the book on a computer. I half-heartedly gave the gentleman my telephone number, thinking that he would not ring, as he probably had not understood my garbled speech. But three hours later he called. I went, consumed by a great feeling of acceptance and euphoria, to pick up the book I had ordered. Since then, I would take the light-writer with me. Instead of giving them my phone number, I gave them my email address.

One day Maya left. Her family needed her in Calcutta. I was left to my own device. I was 30 odd years at the time, but I felt I had not achieved much in terms of my independence. Without Maya, I had a chance of proving myself. I think that is when I began doing things on my own. Actually coming to think of it, my lack of independence first became a source of difficulty during the time of mother's PhD. Mother worked 10 or 12 hours a day.

Yes, I was naturally upset but I feel that carers come and go. I strongly believe that no carer should be regarded as a permanent fixture of life. I was counselling mum and dad as it upset them more than me. I told them that caring for disabled people is not easy and they can get burnt out. There has to be a turnover of carers after a long period.

Without Maya, I began to take on more of the outside work. This was self-imposed. It was, in a way, a relief not to have Maya around. I felt free instead of being constantly forced to be with someone and having to tell someone what to do. Every human being needs space and time on their own to develop and think. If a disabled person is constantly with a person and taken care of, she or he is not going to develop into their own person. My parents praised me and said I was very mature and wise.

Our entertainment and social networking was cut down because Maya was not with us. This helped mother, who focused entirely on completing her PhD. Mother was on a strict deadline and she spent most of her time in the evening working and writing.

One afternoon, a couple of weeks after we moved, dad decided to train me on how to climb stairs using the banisters for support. He felt that I could do it myself. I held onto the banisters like grim death. I was petrified that I might fall, a fear that still dominated me. I have always been apprehensive about doing anything physical that can hurt me. This could be owing to a trigger in an area in the brain that recalls the hurt that was caused at birth with the cord round my neck. Perhaps that made me less forthcoming in doing anything that needs a physical effort. Mother always put it down to 'you are being lazy'.

'Now Molls, hold your two hands onto the banisters and take two steps on to the next step slowly', said dad.

'No, I can't do it', I cried, as he guided me near the staircase. I was petrified. Anxiety overpowered me. I was ready to give up.

'You can do it Molls, just concentrate', he said gently but sternly.

I took one step, and then another, and then I slid my hand gradually down the banister. I had done it ... once ... then again ... and then again. Slowly, I managed to make my way to the stairs. Dad was of course, just behind me. I could feel him every time I took the next step, which helped to bolster my confidence. It soon became relatively easy. Of course it was good exercise.

'Very good', dad said as he gave me a hug. We were both ecstatic. We could not wait to show mother. Mother was ex-ultant and thrilled as she watched me taking the steps. She stood beside me patiently, as I walked down the entire flight of 32 steps. Later, I began to do this task completely on my own when mother was not around.

I was also very independent because of my electric wheel-chair. Every morning, I would get ready and wander around. The whole day stretched before me to explore. I went to librar-ies, bookshops, supermarkets and exhibitions.

'Let's go and see a French film', proposed mother one day.

'Why don't you and Molls go?', suggested dad.

It was easy for mother and me to slip into a cab and reach the cinema hall at Leicester Square. With my electric wheelchair, I did not need anyone to push me. Cinema halls were accessible and my electric wheelchair could easily go into the hall. From then onwards, mother and I went everywhere alone.

My favourite pastime was going to the famous Waterstone Bookshop and reading for hours. I was an avid reader and finished many books. It was at times embarrassing, as I spent hours at the store and the shopkeepers would often give me sharp and stern looks. I read biographies, romances and thrillers. It was such fun, not having to buy, but reading for free.

I was free! Free to go anywhere I wanted. This was very different from the situation in India. It made me forget that I could not walk. Mother was busy writing her PhD. For the first time in my life I was in charge and responsible for my day. It was wonderful to have long stretches of time to myself.

At lunch time, I normally used the Institute's canteen. Within a few weeks, the kitchen staff knew my needs and would serve me my usual order without me even having to ask. I loved fish and chips. The smell of fresh fried fish titillated my taste buds. I often ate lunch alone. Slowly, I ventured out to new places.

'Mother, I am going to have Kentucky Fried Chicken', I said and whizzed off on my wheelchair. I opened the doors of the restaurant with my legs and wheeled up to the queue. Due to my poor speech, the servers could not understand me, so I pointed at two pieces of chicken legs, chips and a coke. The servers came, brought me my order and took the right amount of change, helping me to find a vacant table. So helpful and so unquestioning, I wondered why everyone was not like them. Again, I was consumed by that great feeling of euphoria, which reminded me that I was independent and free!

Despite her rigorous regime that she inflicted on herself to complete her PhD in a short period of time, mother always had time to cook one dish in the evening. Mother was an excellent cook. I strongly believe that being a gourmet cook has its disadvantages as we, as a family, were extremely finicky about what we ate, and poor mother has had to plan endless gourmet meals.

Kaka and Vrinda often came over as they normally visited Europe every year. I decided to show off my knowledge of London and took *kaka* to a Turkish Restaurant on St. James Street.

'Where are we going?', asked *kaka*. 'I am taking you to a cosy restaurant on St. James Street', I said.

Kaka hated walking. He was used to getting into a car and being driven around by a chauffeur. 'Malini, how far is it?' He moaned and groaned, getting impatient.

'I am very impressed by you and how much you know of London', said *kaka*, lighting his cigarette and ordering our drinks.

'You should definitely stay on a few more months in London, as you are so independent here', *kaka* said, one morning; I mustered up the courage and approached mother and pleaded.

Mother had a fixed seat by the PhD. Common Room window, from where she could watch the concourse. She thought that she could keep an eye on my whereabouts but she rarely could. Thank God the use of the mobile phone was not a common practice as yet.

One day, mother said, 'Molls I will teach you how to use an email account'. Mother had just completed a beginner's course in electronic mail use at the Institute of Education. She let me into the PhD Study Room with explicit instructions that I could be thrown out as soon as any PhD student came in. I agreed, and quite often, as students came and went, I had to move away. She logged on to a computer, typed the password and opened a blank page on the computer screen. I typed a short email to my cousin sisters. She then showed me how to type in the address, and with the mouse I clicked 'send'. I did this action two or three times. Within a day or two, I got the hang of it. I acquired a number of email addresses of friends and relatives. I found the computer and Windows software easy to use, and I learnt how to access my email. The email technology revolutionized my life. I was able to communicate on my own. I opened a hotmail account of my own.

Then while mother was busy, I learnt to research on the internet. I could read papers online or could search for jobs or look at what was going on. The internet opened up a whole new world to me. For the first time, I had access to any kind of information. To be able to get any information that I wanted, really empowered me and stimulated my thought processes. I could also communicate with whoever I wanted without requiring a third party. This also empowered my thinking tremendously. And I made friends with students who were studying for their Master's and PhD's and who were closer to my age.

Having mastered the internet and my light-writer, my skills of communication improved vastly. I had my own independent means of communication. This was a kind of freedom from being trapped by my speech impediment and communication difficulties. Seeing my contagious smile and friendly nature (as other's often tell me), I became friends with quite a few people in the Institute. Initially, due to my poor speech, I interacted with them through the internet. Slowly I hung out with them at the IOE Bar, being able to communicate using my light-writer.

They were quite unconcerned about my poor speech. I used my light-writer extensively. I began to grow in my thinking and began forming independent relationships.

During the day, I managed the household chores like laundry and shopping for groceries. For the first time, as a woman, I had a choice of choosing my own things and choosing what I wanted to do, where I wanted to go. I got used to managing the days on my own and doing the shopping, whether it was buying the medicines the family needed, the toiletries, or the cleaning detergents. People in the supermarkets, the chemists and the bookshops, all came forward to help me—something that I had rarely experienced in India.

I must admit I was slightly scared; I was afraid that my wheelchair would break down, or that someone may sense that I was alone and unnecessarily worry about me. If one really thought about it, I had stepped out from my body and the realization of how disabled I really was, because I was totally alone now with speech which was difficult for others to pick up quickly. Yes a million things could go wrong, as mother often warned me, but I was not willing to let my thoughts go down that path. I decided I would worry about these concerns later.

Mother was quite absent-minded. 'Molls, do you want a mince pie?', she asked one day. 'Yes', I said. A minute later we heard a scream followed by a loud noise. Mother ran to the kitchen. The microwave had exploded. She had put the Marks and Spencer's mince pie with the foil into the microwave.

'I think the Microwave has burst', said mother ashamedly, not knowing what had gone wrong. When dad came in, we explained the problem. He examined the microwave. 'Can we fix it?', asked mother. She loved old things and hated buying new things. Dad was the opposite—he loved shopping and never believed in recycling or repairing.

'No, it will cost more to repair. It is better to buy another', said dad. So, the next day dad and I went and bought a new microwave. My wheelchair was always used by us as a 'pull along carrier on wheels'. We put the microwave in a big laundry bag and put it behind my wheelchair and carried it home. The old one was thrown out.

'Molls, we need pasta and cherry tomatoes', said mother one day, as she went off to work after having a quick cup of tea with me. I whizzed off past Russell Square to a Safeway in Brunswick Square. I had such good experiences in the supermarket while shopping. It was unbelievable how helpful people were. Nobody stared. Nobody asked me rude questions. If I could not reach for things, other shoppers would pass me an item. This was so different from India, where they would have come up to me and asked me a million questions, apart from staring at me. The cashiers took out the right amount of change from my purse, never more or never less. They or other shoppers put the bags of shopping on the back of my wheelchair and I whizzed home. It was a good community experience. It made me feel like a contributing member of the family, doing my bit for the house work.

Next, I tackled the launderette. Dad and I usually did the laundry together but on this occasion, he was busy and there was a mountain of dirty clothes that had piled up. 'Don't worry', I said one day. 'Can you put the Laundry Bag on the back of the wheelchair?', I asked mother confidently. Again, there was great resistance. How are you going to take the clothes out? Who will put it into the machine?

I said, 'Please allow me to work this out.'

Thank goodness I had democratic and understanding parents who encouraged me to be as independent as possible, despite some occasional resistance.

I whizzed away on my wheelchair to Brunswick Square Launderette feeling rapturous at the thought of being useful and doing my share of housework. I entered the launderette. The attendant in charge immediately approached me and asked if I needed help. I nodded smilingly. I then went browsing and ran some other errands. Forty-five minutes later I got back to make sure that the clothes were put into the drier. Again, I browsed at the shops as I waited for the clothes to dry. I returned. The attendant again helped. I supervised the folding and had the attendant put it on the back of my wheelchair. Then I was off home.

Slowly, with experiences that encouraged me to be more and more independent, I became bolder!

A Bold French Holiday

'Are you going on a summer holiday this year?', I asked Fiona during one of our long telephone conversations from Bristol to London. Fi and I have known each other since we were toddlers. Our mothers (her mother's name is Janet) were pregnant at the same time; both were living in the steel city of India known as Jamshedpur where my father was based when he was working with Tata. Her parents (the Banes') and we stayed in a huge bungalow with gardens all around. They were called the Kaiser Bungalows. Her father was working with a British company. Our parents soon became close friends. Our mothers were typical ladies of leisure, as they attended the same coffee parties and enjoyed the club culture. Over the years, as the Banes' moved back to England, the friendship progressed as we made routine trips to England and made it a point to visit them in their Solihull house in Birmingham. Fi, too, spent time in India with us.

'A summer holiday? No, I do not have any plans yet', she said.

'Why don't we go somewhere together?', she suggested.

'Sure, why not?', I said unbelievingly.

'Where would you like to go?'

'Paris', slipped out from my lips as if we were playing a game.

'Seriously, let's go', she said.

'Yes, let's go. We will have so much fun'. After I put down the phone, I promptly forgot about our conversation. I could not possibly imagine anyone wanting to take on the challenge of taking me, as well as, the wheelchair, for a holiday.

'Malini, I have found out the price of tickets for a round trip to Paris. Please call me back', was the message left on the answering machine one evening. It was midnight when I heard it. I had gone to see a play, *My Girl*, at the West End theatre with my friend Judith, and then for dinner at a Chinese restaurant in Soho. I had to wait until the morning to get in touch with Fi. I rang her up at 9 o'clock sharp, eager to know what was on her mind.

'If we spend a Saturday night in Paris, it will be cheaper', I said. Both of us had only a few pennies in the bank, but that did not deter us from planning a visit to the most romantic city in the world. So we were going. It seemed as it were a dream.

We made the booking of a hotel through the tour brochure *Access in Paris*. The book proved to be a very worthwhile asset for our holiday. Mother rang up at least 20 hotels and tried to convey in her broken French that the booking required a disabled friendly room with access for a wheelchair.

The day finally arrived. I met Fiona at Heathrow, an hour before the flight was scheduled to take off. Mother advised her never to leave the wheelchair unattended and to always put the brakes on when it was stopped. Fi was amazed to see what special treatment my wheelchair and I received at Heathrow.

'I like travelling with both of you', she said after we got to our seats.

'Ladies would you like Champagne instead of wine?', asked a gorgeous young British Airways steward, who took a liking to us. Seeing the smiles on our faces, he gave us four bottles of Champagne. We opened one, and the rest we put into Fi's big black bag to use as nightcaps. I discovered that Fi's reaction to the intake of wine was similar to mine. A small amount of alcohol would put her spirits on cloud 9. We drove across the city to our hotel, imbibing the beauty of Paris, and nursing the idea of a few glasses of champagne. I was euphoric too, as I could not believe I was in Paris with a friend.

Hotel De France was in the heart of the city, very close to the Latin Quarter in Saint Germaine. Monument Des Invalides, built by Napoleon for the war veterans, was opposite the hotel and its golden gigantic dome served as a landmark for us. The hotel was run by a couple who spoke very little English. 'Bonjour' and 'Au revoir' were the only two words that we said to them daily. We had reserved a double bedroom with a spacious bathroom and a fridge. It served as a comforting and luxurious respite after our hectic days.

Having spent an hour working out our itinerary and examining our map, we walked to the Eiffel Tower. We found the traffic lights confusing. Whenever we crossed the road, our hearts were in our mouths, especially Fi's, whose task was to navigate my wheelchair. At one point my wheelchair nearly went under a car. However, by the last day, she and my wheelchair grew close, as they had devised their own methods of assaulting the French traffic.

Tour D'Eiffel was magnificent. It was thronged with tourists from all over the world. Although the queue was long, it moved quickly. We went up one floor in an overcrowded lift and emerged to see the view of Paris. What a splendid and breathtaking sight. As public transport was inaccessible to the wheelchair, we walked to most places. Fiona had never walked so much in her life. This time our destination was the Louvre. The walk to it was exquisite, alongside the Jardins spread out across Paris, which to me made the city extremely romantic.

We were delighted to discover in our guidebook that the entry to the Louvre was free. Free it may be, but it was initially highly confusing as to where to enter from. But soon our high-powered intelligence equalled that of the French, and we were in. The Louvre was a happening and busy museum. It was massive and was divided into two sections, one for the history of France and its relation to the world, and the other for their world famous art collection. We found their impeccable collection of art through the corridors unending but majestic. Every picture had its own beauty; I wished that I could get postcards of all the paintings so as to keep them in my memory. Hordes of people gathered around with video cameras trying to capture the famous mystical smile of the Mona Lisa. Of course, being a typical tourist, I had to buy a poster of the Mona Lisa before I left the Louvre.

Fatigue set in after five hours. We felt that we had imbibed enough, although we had only seen a quarter of the Louvre. So to refresh our tired bodies, we treated ourselves to lunch at a French café on the banks of River Seine. The atmosphere revived us and then we moved on to the Notre Dame.

When we arrived, the evening service had just finished and the organ was playing in the background. A spirit of euphoria overcame me as we moved around the Church. I had never before seen such beautiful paintings of the Mother and Child. A few priests were busy wrapping up, but they looked as though they were doing it in time to the music. I felt a spiritual presence encircle me. I prayed, and thought about how lucky I had been in life. The memory of the Notre Dame will always be indelible in my mind.

'Smoky time', said Fi, which was her frequent excuse for stopping. This time the halt was on a Pont (bridge), which proved to be an interesting one. Many like us were watching some boys practising roller skating up and down the Pont. Skating was the one thing that I never wished I could do as a child. The skaters were extremely friendly and came up and chatted with us. One of them was so taken up with Fi that he asked her out but Fi declined and hid behind my wheelchair. We were overwhelmed by their friendliness.

Our next halt was at the Latin Quarter. The ambience was European. Cafés were filled with people, young musicians were playing the famous tune of 'dites - moi pourquoi' that brought back memories of my aunt (*mashi*), who used to sing it to me when I was a child. We had a three-course set meal, consisting of a rich, home-made Pate, grilled chicken cooked with white wine, followed by dessert for which we had a mouth-watering mousse A la Chocolate. All this was washed down with a half carafe of Chardonnay, whilst watching and enjoying Parisian life.

Our agenda for the day was not yet over—a boat ride at night was a must. The boat accommodated me with ease. The moon shone on us like a guiding light. The ride was majestic. Paris looked even more beautiful lit up, just as we had imagined.

The last day we splurged a little and bought ingredients for a picnic lunch and plenty of booze. We had a Champagne Picnic at Monument Des Invalides, the nearby park. Fortunately, we did not finish the whole bottle, and instead shared a large mug full.

'Can we take a cab back to the hotel?', pleaded Fi, turning to me as I was controlling the budget.

'Yes but just this once', I said, also feeling a bit high with champagne.

The next day, we took a train to Montmartre and saw Sacre Coeur. Montmartre was full of artists painting detailed portraits. A few came up to us and asked us if we wanted our portraits done, but soon discovered that we were not rich tourists. While sitting there, I thought about Nick and his French girlfriend Alekha, who would often tell me stories about their days in Paris.

The stairs at Sacre Coeur did not prevent us from seeing the church. I managed to walk up the stairs easily. Two tourists helped us lift my wheelchair, but they did not put my wheelchair's brakes on, so she went hurtling down the hundred steps. My poor wheelchair, how embarrassing it was for her, as everybody stopped to see what she was doing and gaped at her, as if it was some sort of entertainment showpiece. Thank goodness I was not on it. The church was certainly worth the climb. We discovered the lift too late, it was pointed out to us by a kindly priest.

Fi had seen a cosy French bistro near the Latin Quarter the night before and was determined to take me there as it looked like it served good authentic French food. We arrived too late, to find the restaurant closed, but we had fallen in love with the area. So we looked around and finally found a quiet Italian restaurant. We ordered spaghetti carbonare and finished a whole bottle of Chianti, while chatting and reflecting on our hectic but exciting three days.

Unfortunately, our holiday ended in a series of disasters.

First the taxi driver took us to Charles De Gaulle airport instead of Orly and charged us double the fare. Fi was on the verge of giving him a sock on his face, which I somehow had to prevent. Luckily we had saved some money which we threw at him with utter chagrin.

The second disaster was our plane at Orly Airport, which was facing engine trouble. We were kept waiting for over two hours. We tried our best to remain calm and patient, as all had gone well so far without a hitch. At last there was an announcement saying, 'certain passengers whose names will be called out will be transferred on to another flight'. Our names were not on the list. Panic set in but within 10 minutes a steward came and rescued us and upgraded us to club class. Although we eventually got to Heathrow, it was a couple of hours late. Mother was waiting, quite frantic.

Then the next disaster occurred. We found out that our bags had been left behind.

'You will get them within a day', the British Airways hostess smiled and said quite nonchalantly. The only trouble was my four bottles of wine were in Fiona's bags and Fiona was going to Portugal, which is where her bags were to be delivered. I lost a few nights of sleep worrying about whether I would get my French wine. Two weeks later my wine arrived. Two weeks. Imagine the sleep I had to catch up on.

For me, it was a unique holiday. It was the first time in my whole 28 years that someone (apart from my immediate family) had had the courage to take me in my wheelchair out for a holiday. My spirits soared. I felt like a bird out of a cage. What a most memorable time under the bridges of Paris, 'down by the river Seine'.

Empowerment in Academia

I was becoming more and more independent. I was managing my own chores, my own shopping, my own social interactions—I was free, and not dependent on others around me. I felt empowered and was keen to face new challenges.

It was mid-November 1998. The academic term began in September, but the Institute wanted to enrol as many foreign students as they could, even if it was a little later in the term. Foreign students brought in more income, as they were required to pay thrice the fee a domestic student did. The Institute was flooded with Japanese students. When they saw me, they would often bow down. It was a polite gesture.

'What does Malini want to do and like to do with her life?' said Anne, an academic friend of mother's. 'Would Malini like to study about the empowerment of women?' Anne asked. 'Do you think she would feel more empowered if she did the Master's in Gender Studies? This focuses on women, their issues, their challenges, and strengthening their beliefs through a study of well known feminist's theories', she said.

'I will ask her, I think she would be interested', mother said.

'How about studying again, Malini?', said mother as we strolled through Russell Square.

I was now more adept on the computer. My power of communication had improved considerably. My one little finger was a powerhouse of strength. I used email all the time. To me, the email and the light-writer boosted my confidence. They were 'my voice' which was scarcely heard. My speed on the computer had increased tremendously. I interacted a lot with my parents and friends. They took time to listen, and valued what I had to say. My opinion was asked for on many issues and people treated me as an equal. Also, London being such a cerebral country, one is constantly learning something new, through the radio, television, the newspapers and the people around. There is not a more intellectually stimulating place than London.

After reading extensively about disabled people coming to the forefront of things and taking up the fight for their own rights, themselves, mother began questioning me on what I really wanted to do. Also, being in the company of MA and PhD students spurred me on to thinking that perhaps I could manage the Master's with my one little finger. I cannot go up and down London aimlessly forever, I thought.

'Do you think I can?' I said anxiously. Given a chance, I could but try; the worst scenario is that I would not be admitted or that I would fail.

The chance came soon. An interview was set up for me at 4 o'clock with Professor Diana Leonard, the head of Women's Studies at the Institute of Education. As I wheeled myself along the familiar Institute's corridors, I felt hugely nervous of whether the professors would understand me. My dysarthric speech would surely be a deterrent. I would be compared to the 'normal' student by a yardstick that judged the conversations they made and how articulate they were. I would surely fail with such a comparison.

We knocked at the door, mother and I.

'Hi', said Diana. 'This is my colleague, Debbie'. They both stood up and shook hands with me.

Diana Leonard and Debbie Epstein were in their early fifties. Both of them were prolific writers, reputed and distinguished academics, who focused on women's issues. Diana's special area of research was 'Women's work at home' which was a form of work that went unrecognized. Debbie's area of interest was 'gender and sexuality and why some women's sexuality is hidden'.

I noticed that both Diana and Debbie were very sensitive toward me. They listened to my speech attentively. They asked me a couple of questions. 'Why do you want to do Women's Studies?' 'Have you read any books pertaining to women?'

I mentioned a couple of books by women writers, which seemed to impress them. The interview lasted 15 minutes. I used my voice synthesizer as much as possible throughout the interview. Finally, they told me that they would let me know. For two weeks, I was on tenterhooks. Then finally one morning, a letter arrived. Dad usually came in from the gym with the post.

'Molls, there is a letter from the Institute, if you wait for five minutes, I will make myself a cup of tea, and open the letter', said dad.

Those five minutes seemed like five hours, as I anxiously waited for dad to open the letter. He pottered around endlessly, making his tea. I was sipping my mug of tea, but my eyes followed his movements. My stomach churned. I was convinced that it was going to be another rejection letter.

'Now lets see', he said, as he took out his gold plated letter opener, which I recently gifted him for his birthday, and read out,

Dear Ms Chib,

I take the opportunity to inform you that you have been granted admission to the Master's Programme.

I was stunned for a few minutes.

'C O N G R A T U L A T I O N S!', said both mother and dad as they hugged me. We were all ecstatic. We soon passed on the message to Nikhil.

'We must get a scholarship', said mother in her usual practical way. She always said this.

'Yes', I readily agreed.

I told my friends Charmaine, who was from Malta, and Gregg, who was from America.

'Hi', I said to Gregg, as I got into my electric wheelchair. Gregg was in the middle of completing his Master's dissertation. Gregg and I had long heated discussions about the social model, society and people.

I showed him the letter.

'Good for you, but it's a lot of hard work', said Gregg casually.

'I know. It will need a lot of work and writing. I hope I will be able to do it', I said apprehensively.

'You will need more time', said Gregg practically. 'See, you need to look into the *Students with Disabilities* document published by the Institute of Education', he suggested, 'I am going to Manhattan to have breakfast. Are you coming?'

'Yes', I said, welcoming the idea of a cup of tea. Manhattan was a quaint little coffee place on Woburn Place. We sat down. He ordered his usual of salmon and a cream cheese bagel.

'How can you eat this day in and day out?' I teased him constantly.

After eating, he opened his bag and showed me a book.

'See, but don't touch'. He thrust the book in front of my face. The book was *Disability Politics: Understanding Our Past, Changing Our Future* by Jane Campbell and Mike Oliver.

'Please can I borrow it?' I pleaded. I was very interested to know more about the recent change in the disability movement.

Gregg had more money than me. He bought a lot of books. I had slowly begun borrowing them and read most of his books. Through reading the current literature on disability, my empowerment began.

'Please?', I said.

'Will you promise to return it?', he asked.

'Of course, don't I always return them?', I said innocently.

'No you don't', said Gregg, pretending to be stern.

'Yes, I know, but you always come to take them', I said.

Later, we found out, that I was to be classified as an overseas student but I was not eligible to do a part-time Master's as international students cannot do a part-time Master's. How incongruous is the economics of it—a foreign student in a four-year programme obviously brought in more revenue. Was there any thinking here?

That evening, we had a family meeting. I revealed what Gregg had mentioned.

'There is no way that Molls can do the Master's in one year. Her speed is too slow', said mother as she sipped her cup of tea.

'We need to ask the University authorities to allow you to do it for four years', said mother.

'This is outrageous, it is unreasonable to expect Molls to complete her Masters in one year', said my tutor, Professor

Diana Leonard in her clipped British accent. (Diana had a PhD from Cambridge).

'I will write to Mr Ward saying that there is no way that Molls can do her Master's in one year.' Mr Ward was the Deputy Director of the Institute. Emails went back and forth from Diana to Mr Ward. Finally the battle was won.

I got a call on a July morning in 1998 at 9 o'clock.

'Hello Molls, can you please come and see me as soon as possible?', said Diana.

I got ready as quickly as I could and went to Diana's office. I wondered what could be wrong. I always imagined the worst. Has my Master's admission been refused?

'Molls, come in', said Diana, opening the door and making space for my wheelchair.

'This came from Mr Ward', Diana said and showed me the letter.

The letter said,

Dear Diana,
The Institute has granted Ms Chib to do her Master's over four years.
Yours sincerely,
David Ward

'Isn't it great?', said Diana.

'Wow, I am so thrilled, thank you very much. You have done everything', I said, beaming.

'It's going to be a lot of hard work', Diana said as I left her room.

'Yes I know, but thank you for believing in me', I said nervously.

The battle was by no means over. The next obstacle was accommodation.

'Where are you going to live?', said Jane one afternoon as we strolled through Russell Square. Jane and I were good friends; Jane worked in the Student's Registry.

'You know that the Institute won't give you accommodation?', Jane said.

'Why?', I asked.

'The Institute doesn't offer accommodation to part-time students', said Jane quite matter-of-factly. Jane was one of those Britisher's who were sticklers for rules.

The next day Jane and I met at Russell Square for a cup of tea. My desire to be independent was so great, that I checked out every student accommodation hall, making my way to each on my wheelchair. I went to every hostel in the vicinity, the YWCA and other such halls. Some places had disabled friendly rooms but the answer was always negative.

'You can't stay in the hall alone due to fire hazard and your disability.' Everywhere I went I suffered acute discrimination.

'Why don't you stay in a Care Home? They will look after you. The Institute will not take any responsibility for you in the Halls of Residence because you are a *disabled student.* You need specialized housing, specialized care and special handling. Why not try Leonard Cheshire home?', said Jane.

I was absolutely appalled. Was this England?

After being so independent, there was no way I was going to be in a care home.

It upset me a great deal and immediately I went and told Gregg. This was the downside of how disabled people were treated here; everything had to be special and costly.

'You know she's right, unfortunately', said Gregg. 'They haven't got their act together.'

Although London was so accessible physically, systems were not in place in higher education in the late 1990s.

The Institute had no policy in place for students with disabilities, no system of support in areas of accommodation or personal assistance. I was one of the first international students who were disabled. Initially, there was reluctance amongst the higher officials of the Institute wanting to do anything special for me as an individual case. There was a person on the staff dealing with students, but she had many other responsibilities, as she was also the Welfare Officer for the entire Institute's student community. There was nobody working on these two crucial areas of accommodation and personal assistance for a student with a disability.

Once they were informed about the provisions specified in the law of their country, by Gregg and others, the Administration was willing to comply and set up a Committee dealing with issues concerning disabled students.

I applied for the same flat my mother had stayed in. The Administration was not willing to give it to me as a student although earlier I had lived there for five years. I was not entitled to it they said. Now I was a fire hazard. They said something I began to hear everywhere I went. No one was willing to take the responsibility of ensuring, that a disabled person was safe. It showed up the fact that the Institute had not addressed the *Equal Opportunity Policy* and there was no accommodation for a person with a disability.

Gregg had already got himself on practically all student committees of the Institute. He had become the President of the Students Union and kept up the lobby on my behalf. He brought up the topic of accommodation for disabled students and my need to stay in the Institute's accommodation, despite being disabled.

Diana again got involved and wrote some key letters to the Administrator of the Institute. My enrolment and acceptance in the Institute had caused a stir. There was quite a lot of conversation around how the Institute did not have accommodation for disabled students. The lobby helped. Then one day, Gregg knocked on our door on the day of my first lecture.

'It's done, the flat has come through', he said.

'What do you mean?', I asked.

'You have it for four whole years, I just met Mr Ward', he said. Number 14 where we had lived for mother's PhD for five years was now allotted to me. I screamed with joy and gave everybody a hug and immediately wanted to go out and celebrate.

However, there was one condition. The Institute would not be responsible for my safety. I had to get my mother to sign a document saying that my parents were responsible for my safety. The battle was not completely won.

I smiled at the thought of being in Bloomsbury for four more years. I was familiar with the surroundings, the shops were easily accessible and I, with my wheelchair, had become a well-known sight.

My Master's classes began on 1 October 1999. These classes were held in the evening. On the first day of the course, I was asked by my tutors to prepare a brief introduction of myself. Through the voice synthesizer, I described my physical disability. There was a great deal of interest in my story. For the first three seminars, the tutors emailed me the questions and topics that were to be discussed, before hand. This gave me an edge over my peers. It allowed me to prepare. It also made my peers understand that I was a thinking member of the team. In these weekly seminars, the tutors told us that an effective way of learning would be to form reading groups.

One day, as I entered class, I was surprised to see Gregg. 'What! You are here? You didn't tell me you were going to be here', I said. The class was filled with women from all over the world. It was hugely multi-cultural. There were women from South Africa, Mexico and Japan and of course from England. Gregg clearly stood out.

'I am taking it as I am working on a chapter on identity for my PhD', said Gregg.

The tutors divided the class up into groups of four or six. This was a key strategy, which they often made use of. It makes students grasp a concept thoroughly. I was lucky that I was in a group of four where we could contribute our thoughts on every essay that we were given to read. In my group, there was Miriam, Anita and Helen, my friends, all patiently listening to what I was going to say. I *can* contribute if people are willing to listen to my monotone.

As I was not experienced in discussing contents of the subjects, my first tutorial was a disappointment. I think my tutors were shocked at how little I understood.

'Why don't you talk to your classmates?', Debbie gently encouraged me.

On reflecting, I think this was the first time I had peers who would listen to my speech painstakingly and respond. Working in a team certainly helped as we could clarify and bounce back ideas on each other. What played a crucial part was that all three of my tutors had an interest in inclusive education and in me. Having a background in inclusive education, they pushed others to listen to me, and pushed me to contribute meaningfully to make intellectual sense. This made me an active contributor of the class. Thus began my academic journey where my voice was heard and what I had to say was important for the first time in my life.

This is vital for people who have speech problems; otherwise they sit passively in a class, not engaging, or interacting with the class on an intellectual level. I had missed out this form of interaction at Xavier's and at Oxford Polytechnic.

Living in the campus was wonderful. I had no way of being silent. I met all my peers in class as well as socially and they soon got to know how to understand me.

'Why don't we meet at 9 o'clock for coffee?', said Miriam.

'Great! Let's have coffee up in my flat', I said. Miriam, Helen and Anita came over and we tried to deconstruct the texts. The texts that we had to read and understand were hard. The style in which they were written was at the Master's level. I spent hours in the library trying to absorb the texts.

Slowly I shed my embarrassment and shyness of not being able to speak the Queen's English and began to speak in class. I began vocalizing and recounting little stories of how people oppress me and discriminate against me.

Although we talked about independence and the social model, clearly again, society had not grasped it and was not willing to accept me as I was. Once as I entered the lift I said, 'Six please'. Looking very alarmed, the lady quizzed, *'Are you alone? Where's your helper?'* I shook my head and luckily for me the lift stopped at my floor and I whizzed out before the lady could say anything. I had done this several times before during mother's PhD, and no one had ever questioned me. When I reached my classroom, I regaled the incident. My classmates and Diana were furious.

On another occasion, I decided to go to the University canteen known as University College London (UCL) for lunch. I went in and stood in the long queue. There were throngs of fresher's all in line queuing up for food. I took my cutlery and was waiting my turn to be served. In my mind, I thought maybe I was going to experience some difficulty in communicating what I wanted, but I went along with the crowd to see what happens. A young man in his thirties came up to me and offered his help.

He turned to me and said, 'Can I help you?'

I accepted it with alacrity. He ordered a chicken korma and chips for himself.

'The same for me', I said, and also gestured as it was on the board. The young man told me to go and sit while he got the food. I found a table. The food arrived. I managed to tell him to cut it up. When I believed all was well, his companion arrived. She was awful; she was very rude.

She came up to the table and ignoring me said, 'How is she alone? She can't be alone as she doesn't know her mind. I have worked with these type of people before. These people do not know their mind, they are mental.' She was young, quite attractive, wearing jeans and a T-shirt.

'Who are you with?', said the man, anxiously. He had been so kind. He was in his late thirties. I gestured to him in between mouthfuls to please go and sit with his friends.

'Who is with you?', the girl asked again.

'I am on my own', I said with great conviction but it was useless.

'Can I see your bag?' She asked me loudly, as if I was deaf.

'No you can't', I said. I really felt like an old woman who refuses to part with her bag. There was something about not wanting to part with one's bag; it was like someone taking your independence.

'I am okay. Please don't worry. I am fine on my own', I said forcefully, but it was pointless, as she obviously did not understand my speech.

'I am going to call the management', the bossy girl said to her man friend forcefully.

Reluctantly, I let go of my bag and took out my purse. My purse had only the cards of my Bombay address, which was probably a good thing.

'Are you a writer?', asked the man.

'Yes', I said.

At last I thought that they had understood that I had not got a mental problem. I ate a few mouthfuls and thought all was fine with the world, but not for long. Miss Bossy Chops returned.

'I am going to go call the management. I know what these people are like, they don't know their minds', she repeated. 'Someone must be with her. She can't be on her own. I have worked with these mental people. It can be very dangerous', the girl said, as she got up. One of the UCL security guards with his radiophone came with the girl.

'No one has reported her missing', the security man said, 'but we will look after her'. With that, she made her exit. The security guard hovered around but soon left realizing I was just finishing my lunch. What a traumatic episode. I had been living in the Institute's premises for over five years, where I had become quite well-known. Nobody had been so offensive. There was nothing I could do but grin and bear it. I never went to UCL again.

I related the episode to my friends that evening. 'Society here is so used to seeing disabled people being accompanied by their attendants. They did not know what to do with someone like you who was unaccompanied and needed help', analyzed Gregg. My friends, Diana and my parents were furious when I told them.

After reading extensively, I found my niche. I began to intermingle episodes of my life with feminist theories. It was to see my own life as compared to non-disabled women. For one of the seminars, the topic was difference and diversity. The word 'difference' is being used to describe the difference between women themselves as well as differences between the two genders. Initially, Women's Studies implicitly was meant for only white, middle class, heterosexual, able-bodied, western women. Women's Studies previously did not explore women from different classes, ethnicities, colour, disability, sexual preference and age. The course enabled me to discover more about myself as a disabled woman. I read more and learnt how disabled women were disempowered. My tutors Diana Leonard, Debbie Epstein, Elaine Unterhalter, Jenny Corbett and Eva Garmanikow gave me the confidence to question what I did not understand. They also motivated me to read more on *women with disability* and wanted to know about my experiences as a disabled woman. I started talking and asking questions in class. It was the first time in my academic life in Higher Education that I had a one-to-one independent relationship with my tutors. They got to know and understand my speech. The system of teaching was very informal. It was more of discussion and of course we were put into small groups. Being in a small group, I talked and participated more.

During my first year, Diana Leonard organized a meeting of all the faculties at the Institute in which I was going to be participating. The library and the computer centre began to be particularly attentive to my needs.

In the four years of my stay, there was a change in attitudes. Modifications were made to the stairs, which were not accessible; a stair lift was put in making the canteen and the bar accessible. These changes were implemented for one student ... me. I remembered the terrible times I had in India with no ramps, no toilets or access to libraries and the canteen in St Xavier's.

As the course progressed, I focused on my individual experiences as a disabled woman. I identified with the writings of an author called Jenny Morris, who was a leading disabled feminist in Britain. I agreed with some of her theories. Before Morris became disabled at the age of 21, she was actively involved in the Women's movement and the Labour movement. Trying to make sense of her new identity as a disabled woman, she put her own personal experience into a broader framework, thus making it political in keeping with one of the central themes of feminism, that 'personal is political'. By 'personal is political', she referred to how a disabled woman copes in her everyday life and the relationship of this with the outside world. A disabled woman might need help with personal care, housekeeping, support with childcare and a number of other responsibilities that a non-disabled woman would take for granted. This did not mean that it was her private individual problem. Society and State needed to address this. As without the help and support of Care staff, disabled people would just have to stay at home.

Personal is public. What well-known feminists with disabilities have done is to publicize their own personal experience and put them in a wider context. This wider context makes *personal assistance* a matter of social concern, a social issue rather than a *private and individual* one. A disabled person must have a professional life. The amount of personal assistance would be decided by the Social Services. Again, if there are no disabled-friendly toilets in a public place where disabled people visit, the issue becomes public impinging and restricting a disabled person's life. These issues concerning disabled people are not merely *individual and personal,* they are public issues, which need to be politicized.

If there is no ramp in certain places, it is not a personal problem, but a larger problem which affects all disabled people, not only me. Having access in certain places is crucial not only for disabled people but mothers who have small children in prams, senior citizens, people who have just had accidents, et cetera.

Other feminists also suggest that being both disabled and a woman, is a 'double disadvantage', which means that women with disabilities have to struggle with the oppression of being a woman in a male-dominated society, as well as the oppression of being disabled in a society which is dominated by able-bodied people. Through reading, I found out that there was a cultural association to disability with dependency, child-likeness and helplessness. A disabled man on the other hand is viewed as a wounded 'male' while a disabled woman is not able to fulfil the cultural expectations. She suffers again due to the cultural stereotypes associated with women being caregivers.

Even the media portrays that the common role of most women is of a primary caregiver in a family. A woman needs to have characteristics of nurturance, warmth, tenderness and compassion. Other duties that a woman is required to perform include child-care, spouse-care, cooking, feeding, soothing, nurturing a relationship and patching up tiffs within the family system. The stereotypical thinking is that women with disabilities are unable to provide this kind of nurturance for a man, nor are they able to satisfy his sexual and emotional needs. I have noticed that it is easier for a disabled man to get an able-bodied partner because society is conditioned to having and seeing women doing most of the house work; it is unheard of men doing all the housework or being positioned as a carer.

I also learnt about the '*body beautiful*' concept. Traditionally, women are only considered to look beautiful and that is it. Most men desire their women to be attractive and beautiful. As far as a disabled woman is concerned, she always gets unnoticed because her body is different. An American feminist writer and researcher, Susan Rendall has called it a '*rejected body*'. Thoughts that occurred to me at that time were about some of my failed relationships with men. They must have only seen my body and rejected me.

I have had a hard time accepting that I am trapped in a rejected body. A body that is not sexually attractive. Some people argue whether sex is that important? Well, in Xavier's I have studied psychology. Sex is a basic physiological need that even animals have. Like any other person my age, I adore romances. Being in the mainstream of life, one sees a lot of images of a man and a woman together. As I grew older, I naturally desired sex and a relationship. Like most women, sometimes I craved to be in the arms of a man. Most men look at me as asexual.

I actually found that society also assumes that disabled women should not have sexual urges, should not even think about sex. How dare we let our thoughts go that way? What an indication of deviance! Society thinks that it is enough to include disabled people but what about including their physical and emotional needs?

It is crazy but society on one hand thinks that disabled people should lead normal lives, but when it comes to the crunch of having an intimae relationship with a person who is disabled, they get scared and pretend that the problem is not theirs. The thought of having an intimate relationship with someone who is different does not even cross their minds. Disabled people are often kept at a distance, as the so-called normal people think that becoming involved with a disabled person would be an onerous situation.

My article 'No Sex Please, You're Disabled', in the *Metropolis* on Saturday, September 1996 had alerted the public that people with disabilities were not children anymore; we had thoughts too, which could be adult thoughts, desires, feelings, passions and expectations like any other non-disabled person.

Like everyone else, I did have the desire for sex. Once when I brought up the subject, people around me started whispering and I was told *'why would you need sex?'*

That was the reaction of some of those who called themselves professionals of the Spastics Society. I thought of how they lived in tiny boxes and how small their spaces were. I promptly wrote an article 'No Sex Please, You're Disabled' a take off from a famous comedy I had seen in London of *'No sex please we are British!'* Did it make an impact? I do not think so.

I did have outbursts as, at times, I found life extremely painful. During those moments, I collapsed in tears but I always chose the night and cried quietly. My mother says if she asked me why I was crying I would usually say, 'you know why'. She too would go away and cry.

When I am in an emotional state, I cannot figure why the tears keep rolling down; I cannot control them. Of course, I have normal desires that are hidden and left in a box with a lid never to be opened. But sometimes, the lid slips open and the tears are let loose. It is but natural that I ask myself 'will I be like everyone else? Will I be normal?'

It needs a lot of grit and determination to be different and stand out. I am determined to fight and win! The positive side in me takes over and I keep those painful thoughts away from plaguing me.

One such episode occurred after I returned from my cousin Aditi's wedding to Khalid. I was staying with *kaka* and Vrinda. I collapsed into floods of tears, for no apparent reason. After an age, my uncontrollable tears stopped and I tried to verbalize my emotional outbursts of needing a partner, like most people around me. Both Vrinda and *kaka*, poor things were shocked and did not know what to do or say.

'Yes I agree with you. You should satisfy your sexual needs', said Vrinda.

But of course no one knew how?

Weddings tended to have that affect on me as they were a reminder that I possibly would not ever share such an equation with someone.

I must say I was better during my brother Nicky's wedding to Natasha. I had become more detached. I did not anymore think the only way forward was marriage. Also Natasha (now of course my good friend) being American, having been exposed to disability much more than an Indian woman, is very inclusive. She includes me automatically, not needing to be prompted.

As time progressed, I began developing a close emotional relationship with a close male friend online.

The other thought that I learnt and of course experienced is that disabled people are looked down upon as a burden on society. Susan Wendell writes that any society despises an adult who needs help to eat, wash and to use the toilet. She also goes on to say how the same culture promotes the self-deception that 'independent' adults do not need another's help and ignore the thinking that we are all profoundly dependent on one another.

Everyone is inter-dependent. If one lives in a family for example (be it if one has a disability or not), we are all in a way inter-dependent or co-dependent—socially, emotionally, physically and intellectually. Are not we dependent on the plumber, the electrician, the computer technician?

To give my own example, while my mother was doing her doctorate, we used to share the household chores. While I did all the outside chores, like the shopping, the laundry, posting letters, she did all the cooking and cleaning of the house. We were both co-dependent. She was dependent on me, little old me! In my opinion, to ignore this factor of co-dependency would be to move towards a most self-centred, self-focused world and ignore the support that people like me give.

I buried myself into the Master's Programme. As I kept reading and discussing concepts during my Master's, it gave me more confidence and self-esteem. It was the best time of my life. This was the first time I was analyzing myself and the outside world. I got the opportunity of developing a wide circle of friends and having deep relationships with women the same age as me. Some of them are Miriam Mareso, Patricia Smith, Anita Mathur, Kamela Usmani, Katya Burton, Helen Poulson and of course Susan Kearney, who is my closest friend. All of them were very keen about their careers; they did not come from a male dominated society. By interacting with them, I was able to broaden my knowledge and enrich my life.

With 'feminism' came the understanding that it is crucial to start from the knowledge of our everyday experiences to develop a broader picture and understanding of the oppression of women. This expanded to a recognition that this applies not only to generic 'women's oppression' but also to the different experiences and ways in which different groups of women—including *women with disabilities*—are oppressed. Living on one's own with friends, being accepted for what I am and learning, boosted my confidence and empowered me. It made me believe in myself that I *can* be included in the mainstream of life, *despite* my disability.

My one small finger did not let me down. I became quite adept and fast in writing essays and keeping to deadlines. Only it was slow and laborious. I found the four years intellectually invigorating and emotionally empowering. Were it not for my friend Gregg, and my mentor and guru Diana, I would not have gone through this meaningful and stimulating period which brought me to the crossroads of life, as I began to question myself in terms of who was I? I was, for the first time, able to accept my own identity as *a disabled woman*, and was *proud* of being one.

Living on One's Own

My road to independence and living alone started when I came back to London with my mother in 1996. I was able to master the daily chores as everything was so accessible and everybody around was eager to help.

'Klaus has invited us for a weekend', said mother one day, stirring the pasta sauce.

'Why don't we go?', dad asked.

'Please, can I stay on my own?', I pleaded.

'You can't stay alone', mother said promptly.

'My friends, Helen and Keith are coming. I will ask them to stay on a little longer', I said confidently. Helen and I had gotten to know each other in Oxford. She used to teach at the Polytechnic. After we were introduced, it did not take us long to become good friends. Helen was a poet.

'How do you know if they want to spend the entire weekend with you?' mother inquired.

'I will find out', I said. I dialled their number.

'Hello', said Helen.

'Hello, Helen. It's me, Molls. Mithu and Sathi are going away this weekend. Would you like to come and spend the weekend in London?' I asked.

'We'd love to', said Helen, sounding very pleased. Mother was hovering near the phone.

'Can I speak to her?', asked mother, not trusting that Helen had gotten the right message. I handed the phone to mother. 'Hi Helen, Sathi and I are going off for the weekend and Malini was wondering if you would like to spend the weekend with her here in London?'

Do parents realize how over-protective they are?

'Yes, we would love to', said Helen.

'Then what time do you think you will come?', asked mother.

'We will come by 6 o'clock', said Helen.

'Where will you meet them?', asked mother, as usual anxious and micro managing.

'Don't worry, I'll send them an email and will meet them at the Institute foyer', I said.

'Okay, that seems to be a good arrangement', said mother. I uttered a shriek of joy. This is very characteristic of me. When I am pleased, I shriek with delight. For the first time, I was going to be alone in London with my friends.

On Saturday night, we decided to stay in, watch a video and experiment with our cooking techniques.

'Molls, where's the oven switch?', Helen asked.

'It should be there', I said getting up in my walker trying to look, but failing to locate it.

These are practicalities I had no knowledge of.

'Keith, can you come here and help us find the oven switch?', commanded Helen.

Helen was essentially a feminist but a great householder. Poor Keith was enjoying a few minutes away from the ladies, reading the newspaper.

'Okay coming', said Keith.

It took us the next 15 minutes to find the switch. This was a completely new learning task for me.

'Dinner is ready', said Helen.

We had a lamb casserole, garlic bread and salad, not to miss a bottle of Chianti. For dessert we had a lemon meringue pie.

When we were going to bed, I thanked Helen.

'Wouldn't you do the same for me?' she said as she helped me put on my pajamas. I nodded and would always remember our conversation.

We had a lovely weekend.

My mother and dad looked extremely refreshed when they returned. Must make them get away more often, I thought. I was happy that they were back but glad that I had had some time alone with my friends.

Soon I had another occasion to be alone.

Mother and dad were needed in India. They would be gone for six weeks. It was pointless for me to go and come back. It was also too expensive. It was the monsoon season in Bombay and after my newly found freedom I found the thought of going back to India unappealing as I would be trapped at home most of the time.

'Mother please, I will be able to manage. Let me stay in London on my own.'

This was a difficult request for my mother. Most of the time that I spent away from them was carefully structured and to leave me alone in London was not going to be possible.

'What if something happened to you? What if you became ill?' mother said.

'Nothing will happen to me. Don't assume the worst', I begged. I could be very obstinate and once I made up my mind, I hated to budge from my decision, one of my disabilities among many.

'Let's see', said mother as she ironed some of our clothes. The conversation for the next few days always centred around the subject of whether I was or was not to be left alone in London.

Two weeks later dad asked mother, 'Darling, how many tickets shall I book?'

'I think two. Molls is very keen to stay and we have to respect her wishes.' Mother was essentially hugely democratic (though she loved structure and organization). On hearing this, I instantly gave her a big hug.

This time, I asked my friend Claire to stay with me. She came over to discuss her stay with me. The previous night, mother had cooked a vegetarian meal. Claire loved Indian *khana* (food in Hindi). Claire and I had met through our mothers who were good friends. Her brother Charles also had cerebral palsy like me and coincidentally we were in the same school, both in Cheyne and Delarue. While we were in Cheyne our mothers, Shirley and Mithu, became close friends. When we returned to England this time, we met up after 20 years. They re-introduced Claire and me. When Claire and I met, we bonded immediately and became good friends. It was at this time Claire was forming a group called 'Project Discover'. The aim of this group was to create a virtual environment for disabled people. She and I spent hours working on proposals.

At the dinner table, as we discussed the details of Claire staying with me, mother repeatedly asked, 'Will you be able to manage alone?' We both assured her that we would.

The day arrived for mother and dad to depart. 'Will you be okay?', asked mother for the tenth time as she put her last essentials in her suitcase. 'Yes, of course', I assured her.

By that time, I was trying to keep a brave face.

We walked down the stairs. I was painfully slow as it is, but today I was doubly slow, as I was a bit on the teary side. I guess when one is emotional their balance gets slightly affected.

'Bye', said dad as he kissed me, adding 'this is what you wanted, so don't cry'. Men do not understand why women cry.

'Bye', said mother through her tears, as she hugged me goodbye. Her dark glasses were on. She always put them on when she cried.

The mini cab drove off to Heathrow Airport. To sooth my emotions, much like the English do, I indulged in a cup of tea. I found a café at Russell Square where I sat quietly and dried my eyes. A mixture of emotions passed through me. I was happy to be finally on my own, but sad that my mother and dad had left. We did so much together. We were more like friends.

As I zoomed around on my own, I met so many different kinds of people. People usually would come up to help or to converse which, though on a superficial level, made me feel good as I felt included.

After my cup of tea at Russell Square I decided to check my email. 'Are you a student?', asked an attractive Asian girl. I was searching for a computer to do some internet browsing. It was August. All computers were occupied as the MA students needed to complete their dissertation.

'No', I confessed.

'Then what are you doing here?', she said trying to be fierce.

'My mother is doing her PhD and I wanted to use a computer', I said shyly. 'These computers are *only* meant for students', she said. I gave her one of my sweet, angelic smiles.

'Okay. Just this once', she said.

'What's your name?', I asked.

'Kamela. Yours?', she said.

It was through such interactions that I came to know more and more people, which served to reinforce my independence. I realized that I need not be so apprehensive of managing without mother and dad and that I would be just fine.

Claire moved in that evening.

One evening, Claire asked me, 'Molls, who does the laundry?'

'I do it normally', I said.

I told Stella, my carer, to put the laundry bag on my wheelchair and I whizzed off to Brunswick Square. I dumped the laundry and easily found someone to help me put all the laundry into the washing machine. I told Claire about this.

'I am impressed', Claire said as she came in from work.

For my care, I had two people—one came in the morning and helped me with my bath and getting ready and the other came in the evening to help with dinner.

For the first time, I had to cook for myself as my evening carer came from Nigeria and knew how to make only Nigerian food. I used to tell my carer what I wanted and how to make it, by telling her exactly what to put into the dishes. It was a step-by-step cooking process and she greatly enjoyed it. My cooking was not great, but it was edible. I made meat sauce and pasta on a regular basis in those days. Pasta was considered to be a wholesome, student-friendly of meal.

'Let's have a party', said Claire one day.

'Okay', I said.

It was the end of summer. We managed to squeeze in about 30 people in our small flat.

'Shall we open another bottle of wine?' suggested Claire. It was about 10.30 pm. We felt we had not had enough so we opened another bottle. It was a disastrous decision. We both took two or three sips and got hopelessly sick all over the carpet. Our intake of alcohol was obviously a trifle too high. The tedious task was to quickly remove the stain and the smell.

Six weeks passed without any hassle and I managed just fine. Mother and dad returned from India and we soon settled back into our routine.

Unfortunately, soon afterward, my aunt got very sick, and mother had to return to India again. Dad was in Bombay at the time.

'Molls, *mashi* is in intensive care', mother informed me as I sat down.

Mashi was my aunt's sister. *Mashi* and my relationship goes back to the day I was born. When I was born apparently I spent a significant amount of time with her. When we moved to Cambridge, she helped mother to take care of me. Until I was 22 I did not have a carer. My personal needs were taken care of by my mother and members of the family. As my mother and my aunt were getting older, *mashi* only suggested that I should have a separate carer. Her stroke was a big and tremendous tragedy in our lives.

Mother's face was red as she had been crying. Her eyes had dark circles too as she had limited hours of sleep since she came back from India. She had finished her 100,000 words thesis. It was phenomenal as she took only two-and-a-half years to complete her PhD which usually takes a minimum of five years. But her viva was yet to happen.

'You come after the viva', said *mesho*. We spent a fortune on phone calls.

'Ma, don't worry. You go after your viva. I will come a bit later.' I said bravely as I counselled her.

Who will stay with you? mother asked.

'One of my friends, don't worry ... now I am a student, I know quite a few people', I said in my confident way. After all I was now a qualified student. I had nothing to fear. Previously, there was a nagging worry about whether or not I will be asked 'who are you and what are you doing'. As soon as I became a student I got more confident and found out my rights.

'I will find someone', I said. My formula of living alone was to carry on with the carers and have a friend to share the flat. This had worked. So I rang up my friend Charmaine.

Within a day, Charmaine said yes. Mother flew to Delhi after her viva and Charmaine and her sister stayed with me.

'Sweetie, what shall we have for dinner?', said Charmaine.

'Shall we have homemade pizza?'

'Sounds lovely, but how?', said Charmaine.

'I have bought pizza bread and the ingredients. All you need to do is to pop some vegetables on top of the pizza bread and then add the cheese.'

'Don't we put cheese before?', said Charmaine.

'Yes, sorry, my cooking skills are elementary', I confessed as I sipped my wine.

Charmaine prepared the pizza and put it in. The pizza was ready within minutes.

'It looks brilliant', I said as I bit into a piece.

'You have good cooking skills', Charmaine exclaimed.

'So do you', I said, as we chomped on our pizza, very satisfied with life. We patted each other on the back for our successful attempt at homemade pizza.

'Meet me at the Institute of Education (IOE) bar. I am inviting some friends', said Miriam, one of my classmates. Miriam was half Ethiopian and half Italian. Within a couple of weeks, Miriam and I had become good friends.

'Okay', I said, rushing to hurriedly complete some Christmas shopping on Tottenham Court Road as I was leaving for India the next day.

I arrived at the IOE bar with bags in my wheelchair. 'These are my friends, Susan and Kamela', said Miriam. After a while Miriam drifted to another table with her friends.

'You have been doing a great deal of Christmas shopping', said Susan as she noticed a considerable amount of bags at the back of my chair. 'Yes, I am leaving for India tomorrow and these are Christmas presents', I said.

We had a good evening. What was unique about that evening was that we chatted and had a great deal of fun. I think what I intently love about friends is that they first see me as a person and then my disability. This is one of the main reasons why we remained friends for the next 12 years.

When I returned from India in early January, I was alone for a brief period of two weeks. I organized a student every night to come and stay the night with me as the higher officials did not want me to sleep the night alone in case of a fire.

After I returned, I kept bumping into Susan and Kamela at lunch-time. At that time they were both assistants to Professor Angela Little and Elaine Unterhalter, respectively. Susan and Kamela threw a party for the students in their department, to which I was invited.

'Why don't you come for a cup of coffee?', I asked them one day.

'Okay', they said. They came and we ate, chatted and laughed. We discovered that we gelled extremely well, laughed at the same jokes, shared the same interests and liked the same films.

'We are having another party, so we are doing some shopping', they said as I bumped into both of them in Brunswick Square one day.

'I will help you, why don't you put your shopping bags on my wheelchair?', I said.

'A very good idea', said Susan, who liked taking the easy way out. Whenever they had parties, I would go along with them and my wheelchair would carry all the goodies with surplus bottles of wine. Susan and Kamela got attuned to my speech very quickly. I have realized that some people have a quick knack of understanding my speech.

'Are you free on Saturday? Why don't we to go to a movie?', I said to Susan and Kamela.

'I am free. Lets go to Renoir, there's a French film on', said Susan.

'Yes, let us', I said.

So, we went. In those days the Renoir was inaccessible, so Susan helped me walk down the stairs.

As months went by, we became inseparable. Once I had gone in to have a quick chat and a cup of tea during office hours, which they did not encourage; as Professor Little came out to where the offices were located, I made a quick dash. My exit was quite obvious. Being on a wheelchair one can be so conspicuous. There is nothing subtle about me.

All three of us became extremely close.

'I am going to Paris with the students', said Susan, 'do you both want to come?', she asked Miriam and I.

'Yes, I would love to', I said.

When I told dad, he thought about it for a while.

'Well, if Miriam is going, then you can', said dad.

We scheduled a visa appointment at the French embassy for the next available night.

Susan and I booked one of those dial-a-cabs to take us to the French embassy. Unfortunately, we had some bad luck. My electric wheelchair broke down in the middle of the road. I had to convey to Susan where the free wheel was for the electric wheelchair. The situation was dangerous as cars were zooming past us. I think Susan got frightened of using the electric wheelchair. She preferred me in a manual wheelchair.

'What? You girls could not manage to get the visa?', dad said picking me up from the IOE bar.

'No', said Susan. We all grinned to mask our nervousness.

'Okay. I will go tomorrow', he said.

The next day as he walked in through the door I asked, 'Did you get it?'

'Yes, I got it. Unlike you girls, I managed to get it.'

Kamela and I travelled together on the Eurostar. We discovered that Eurostar offered a deal whereby one's carer gets half-price. Both Miriam and Susan were delighted with such a scheme. On arriving in Paris, Kamela and I shared a room with Miriam and were going to meet Susan the next day. Kamela helped me take a shower and get dressed. It was good to give Miriam an extra pair of hands to help look after me. On that trip we had an advantage; Miriam and her brother spoke fluent French. My friends who were vegetarians were shocked when I ordered Frog Legs and shoved slithering snails down my throat.

'Molls, do you really want to eat this?', Susan said. She always hoped that I would become vegetarian.

'Yes, it is delicious. Why don't you have one? Be adventurous', I said to the others. They shook their head and refused. I felt like a carnivore as everyone watched me munch on Frog Legs.

Paris was beautiful and snowy. As we walked around the Notre Dam area, snowflakes fell on us. The holiday was splendid. For me, it was absolutely heavenly and wonderful to be with peers who were my own age.

The Paris holiday was the first of many.

Today, it is an annual practice for us to go somewhere together every year. I usually am the initiator and the organizer. The holiday is decided upon when I hit London for the summer. So far, we have been to Edinburgh, Devon, Uppsala and Goa. We discovered steep hills in Edinburgh and Devon. Both Susan and Kamela pushed my wheelchair up the steep hills together. After that holiday, the poor things needed another one. In Goa we came across the potholes of Baga Beach and the stares of the locals. Either they were gaping at my wheelchair or Susan's body (Susan in her swimsuit was very sexy for the Indians).

I will always cherish my holidays. It is superb to be with people one's own age even for a short time.

As time progressed, I was becoming more and more independent—staying back while my parents travelled, taking holidays with friends. I was glad that I was no longer so dependent on my parents and if need be, they could leave me home alone without worrying about me.

One evening we got another terrible news.

Amma had passed away in June 2001. It was devastating for us. *Amma* was dad's mother. After her husband died, she had led a very independent and empowered life. *Amma* was a professional cook for 40 years. When she became a widow, she fiercely guarded her independence. Dad was very quiet and upset. Nikhil had spoken to him and had taken charge of *amma's* body.

'Molls, I have got a ticket for tomorrow morning at 8. Will you be alright on your own?', dad said.

'Don't worry I will get my friend Katia to come and be with me', I said. Katia lived on campus.

'Are you sure?', asked dad.

Looking back, I realize how significant my new found independence was. Had I not been able to manage on my own, mother and dad would have had the added burden of tending to me at such difficult times.

I rang up my Mexican friend Katia. 'Katia, can you come at five, my parents have to leave for India' and I explained what had happened. Realizing it was an emergency, she came at five in the morning.

'I would also like to tell Greg. I will feel more secure', said dad. As usual he was being overprotective. Sometimes it was irritating but sweet too.

After a day or two Susan moved in. We spent six weeks together. It was a difficult time for the family and Susan and I tried to keep busy and not think about it too often. We went for walks, ate out a great deal and talked at length. In the mornings, the Bee Gees or ABBA was invariably on as we got ready for work. Each day as she left for work, the song 'Tragedy' played, signifying how she felt about work.

One day I asked her, 'Why are you with me most of the time?'

'I like difference. It attracts me.' I had gotten used to living with Susan and, was in a sense, a little sad when dad came back and she had to move out. Emotionally, I was happy with Susan and it was an idyllic period of my life though it was also a difficult time.

My next flat mate was Varsha, my close friend who worked for ADAPT. She had come to London to do her Master's, which was partly from the Institute of Education and partly from a Canadian university. She brought her daughter Simran with her. Simran was five-and-a-half. As I was writing my dissertation, I did not have any classes in the evening. I micromanaged every activity so that she was ready before her mother came back home at night from the library. My first experience of motherhood was in looking after Simran's needs.

What? A Second Master's—Unbelievable!

After the first Master's, working at the Institute's Library was ideal for me. With all the information computerized, one could communicate and interact through the internet and so not very much speaking was needed. Thank goodness for technology for people like me who needed wheelchairs for mobility and computers for communication! I had a special corner which I considered mine. I buried myself for a year in the Library. I had to complete four assignments for the Master's programme, which was the requirement for the University. Each assignment needed an argument which was crucial, a reference to all the current writings on the subjects and a detailed bibliography stating all sources of information. All this with one finger! What people did in an hour, I took an entire day. So, it was nose to the ground hours in front of the computer.

Socially, I did well. Despite my poor speech, I had a knack for networking and making friends easily. I smiled and maintained eye contact and could quickly develop a friendship! As months passed, I had become friends with a few of the library staff.

'Why don't you become a librarian?', said Gwyneth, one of my librarian friends. 'You could come and go whenever convenient. You will have flexible hours.'

'I would love to', I said.

I was told again. 'Why don't you do a course in becoming a librarian? You know Victoria is doing that course next year', said Anne Peters, a good friend, Head of Information Services and the Library at the Institute of Education, very sound in her advice. Anne and I used to regularly meet for a cup of coffee and a chat.

I shared this with my parents. Mother who had been thinking that I needed something more professional said, 'Okay, if that's what you really want to do!'

I was not completely sure myself, so I took a year off. I spent my time in three different Libraries, two of which were in Bombay and one in Canada. I spent a week in the University of Prince Edward Island in which my friend Vianne Timmons was Vice President of the University. While I was in Bombay, I divided my time between the British Council Library and the Library at the American Centre. There was much discussion amongst my inner circle of friends and family whether to do a second Master's or not.

The new buzzword in Library Science is information management. I did not need much speech as most of the information needed was on the World Wide Web.

'Why don't we check out the University of North London?', I said to mother and dad.

The reason I thought of this particular course at the London Metropolitan, University of North London, was because it was the latest course in Librarianship.

We set out to Ladbroke House, next to the Highbury fields in Islington where the London Metropolitan University carried out some of their programmes. It was a cold windy day in April

2005 a trek from Pimlico to North London quite rightly described by Elliot in Wasteland as the 'cruellest month', weatherwise.

I was interviewed by Sue Bately who was the Course Leader and later became my personal tutor. Looking through all the paper work, and my CV (which now looked quite robust!) she said, 'you will have no problem getting in as you have already got a Master's, but fill in the application form. She asked me a few questions and I replied on the voice synthesizer. After a while, she said,

'You are in and we'll send you the formal letter.'

I was allotted a two room flat in Holloway. The Residence known as *The Arcade on Holloway Road* was hugely accessible, different from the IOE. The flat made me really feel free. The toilet was spacious, large enough for a wheelchair to turn around, spacious bedrooms and kitchen. This empowered me further and enabled me to make quick decisions of moving around in the flat itself. I could check what was in the fridge and what I needed to buy. The London Met also had a special Disability Welfare Officer who was hugely attentive to me. The only problem was transport. I had to change two buses to get to my college. I quickly got the knack of getting in and out of the buses. I stayed with a flat mate called Gulab, who stayed with me for three months, taught me how to push and get on to the bus! Initially, I felt scared and reluctant to push my way. It took me a while. For the first few months I always had friends or my mother or Sathi or two flatmates, Varsha and Gulab, accompany me.

'Where have we come?', said mother in her snooty way. She was only used to the posh parts of London. She said, 'This is spectacularly horrible!' Holloway is associated with the famous Holloway Prison. But Holloway grew on me and my friends. We adored the charity shops, the restaurants and a slower pace of life, not like the Institute with its proximity to exciting Bloomsbury.

'Look at what we have here', said Susan as we moved into the Red Bar.

The Red Bar looked pretty atrocious from outside but when we went inside, it was cosy and had blaring music on. The Red Bar served good Thai food right at the doorstep of the Arcade! It had a great atmosphere with lively music. By the end of my stay, the Red Bar became an extension of our drawing room.

'Here, what do you want to eat?' Susan said as she handed me the menu.

Kamela, Susan and I used it a great deal to chill out.

'You will be a good trainer', said Richard Rieser who was in charge of '*Disability, Equality and Education*'. Richard gave me a part-time job, whereby I was in touch with many disabled adults. I was given a personal assistant. I had to learn how to use a personal assistant at work. My job included formulating a database of disability trainers and giving training on disability issues and inclusive education.

At the London Met, I noticed that most students were texting and using a mobile phone. Texting was beyond me because it involved such finite co-ordination, too fiddly for me. But seeing my friends communicate at a fast pace and seeing it does not need speech, I was determined to learn it as it is the quickest way of keeping in touch with friends and family.

'Here are three different mobiles, I will leave them for you to try them out', said our friend Frances Cairncross. Frances and Hamish also gave me a computer so I could work at home. They lived in Islington—a fashionable part of London and hardly ever came to Holloway except now to visit mother and me. My one little finger did not adapt to these mobiles.

It was a Saturday when, after saying goodbye to my friend Sumitra, I decided to go to the Carphone Warehouse—the Mobile Shop. I managed to convey my need to see a couple of mobiles. The shop assistant showed them to me. None of them suited my needs. I left after seeing every mobile! I felt bad at disrupting the shops. After spending ages fiddling around with my Indian mobile at night in my bed, I got it. Poor Susan! I think she got innumerable SMSs in the beginning.

The course at the London Met, was a very professional one. All students were older than me, already in jobs and moving on to be Librarians. The library and information profession was in a period of rapid change. New information and communication technologies have revolutionized the production, storage, retrieval and dissemination of information. The management of information services and the formulation of information policies of the organization are being constantly re-evaluated. We learnt the differences between search engines and web directories. It taught an entire range of different and complex ways of searching from search engines. I also learnt about the various information policies certain organizations have.

The course concentrated more on management styles of functioning within a library, the various different methods of management. It taught me website design, setting up an intranet system. What attracted me to the course was that I had to do a six week placement at any library. I chose LSE, as my friend Victoria worked there and also I went there often when mother was there. I did not think I would get in. I went for an interview with my friend Victoria. It certainly helped to have contacts and friends. I was interviewed by one of her colleagues called Beverley. The interview went well. I communicated with my light-writer! I got the five week placement! I was thrilled that I would have a chance of working in LSE. I secretly hoped that I would get a job after my six weeks of placement. And I got in only using my light-writer! I could see that attitudes towards people with disability were changing, even in the last five years.

The five week placement was tough. I had to wake up at 7 o'clock. It was the heart of English winter! Stella my carer came promptly at 7.30 am, after leaving her home at some unearthly hour to help me get ready. Poor Varsha who was living with me for a term finishing her Master's used to wake up early to help us as time was limited. She would make my lunch snack each day. The English weather made Varsha very depressed, poor thing!

Stella and I would proceed to the bus stop for the good faithful old 91 bus which took us to Holborn and Portugal Street. The frequency of 91 was one in every 10 minutes. Very often, while waiting at the bus stop for the accessible 91 bus, it began to snow. There we would stand under umbrellas with snow around us everywhere! Beautiful, but also physically strenuous.

Varsha would always be prompt at picking me up in the evenings. We made friends on the bus! 'You are a wonderful person', said a passenger on the bus to Varsha as she saw Varsha help me. 'God will bless you'. Varsha and I secretly had a laugh (medical charity model we thought, anyone helping us disabled, would be blessed!).

'Varsha please let me go on the bus on my own. It's easy'.

'There's no way I am going to let you go on the bus on your own', she said. I love Varsha, but she can be obstinate! I felt frustrated that I had someone with me all the time, as much as I like to be with them. I could never meet anyone spontaneously and that depressed me.

There was a short period of time when I had to live on my own as mother needed to go back to India for her work. I was staying with friends, Kamela and Carol, who were students studying at the Institute. They took turns to stay with me. Susan and Kamela were really over-protective and were always ready to pick and drop me. But they had their own lives too. After all, I had mastered crossing the busy roads of Central London. I had the freedom of crossing the roads, why could not I go in and out of buses by myself? The night before it was decided that when my lectures got over the next day I would wait for Kamela to come and pick me up.

Things did not work out according to plan. Classes got over early. I decided to take the plunge and got into the bus on my own! There is a special space on the bus for wheelchairs and prams. The driver on seeing me brought the ramp out electronically. There were always many people around to help me get off and get on. I decided to go to Russell Square (the one area which had been home to me for nine years). It meant taking three buses! There were people in the bus whispering loudly as if I was hard of hearing '*Is she alone?* , or, *How can she be alone?*' I heard two old ladies say: '*I thought them people were not allowed out alone!*' By the time they figured it out, I had reached my destination and indicated to the driver about needing the ramp. I zoomed out in my electric wheelchair, waved goodbye to the driver and proceeded to my destination. Travelling by bus did not need any speech. Being alone was terrific. It allowed me to interact with the community. The experience cut out disability, the everyday experiences which non-disabled people take for granted. I was so used to being driven around by a chauffeur in Bombay and escorted in London. This was so novel, so exciting! I felt fantastic that I could travel on my own.

I started going everywhere on my own, I went and browsed at bookshops at Regents, in Charring Cross or just roamed around old favourite haunts like Russell Square, Regents' Park and Tottenham Court Road. I loved Waterstones, Blackwell and Foyle's, they are my favourite places. I am a familiar figure there and would meet my friends there. Blackwells is my favourite bookshop—it has comfortable lounges and a quaint area where you can finish a whole book and nobody would disturb you!

Previously, friends came to meet me at one venue. Now, I could meet them anywhere! The feeling was great. Euphoric! Unfortunately, I had to learn the bus routes through mistakes! Once I was meeting an old friend in the Russell Square Café, then I had an appointment in Holloway. I took four buses to get to the office, by mistake! My friend Michael Bach, Director of Canadian Association for Community Living (CACL) from Canada met me in Piccadilly and was intrigued and amazed at how well I knew the London buses and how I navigated through the busy West End!

How I loved London! The freedom, independence and acceptance of people like me made me feel alive.

Of course I got many SOSs from home, mainly from my father and brother to say 'please take a cab'.

When my mother returned (she was usually in India but would come frequently for short stays); I slowly broached the subject that I had cracked the London's buses on my own. 'Ma, I will take you on a bus', I said. Yes, she was annoyed but her anger disappeared when she saw me hopping in and out of the buses with ease, and how many came forward to help. My mother had never travelled in a bus! Unbelievable ... she took the underground usually.

'Pretend you don't know me and just observe how well the other passengers help me', I said to mother.

Mother noticed that if the bus driver did not hear my buzz, the fellow passengers would tell the bus driver to stop and take the ramp out and then I would zoom out and wave goodbye to the bus driver and the passengers. This indeed caused a chuckle. Mother and I began going everywhere together on buses!

My two Master's gave me confidence. I had to rely on myself as my friends had full time jobs. I had brought Vimla, my Indian carer, but her knowledge of English was nil. It forced me to do more in London on my own. Why not check the facilities and attitudes toward disabled people further, I thought.

The year at the London Met was very intensive. The assignments needed a lot of work, a lot of reading.

After my Master's in Information Management, I decided to spend the summer looking for a job from our tiny little flat in Pimlico. Our flat is very well situated overlooking the river Thames. Initially, it took me a while to settle down to life in Pimlico. It was a quiet life compared to the campus atmosphere both at the Institute and Holloway, Pimlico being hugely central. I loved it. The Battersea Park was just round the corner. I soon became known in the local shops of Sainsbury, Tesco, the cultural hub which in the South Bank is about 40 minutes walk on the riverfront, a beautiful walk. I generally hung around there browsing through the second-hand books and seeing old French films. I became an avid reader and a member of the local library. I chuckled with joy when I found my favourite romances. My uncle (*mesho*) came for a meeting to London. I took him down the beautiful walk down Grosvenor Road to my old school at Cheyne Walk.

I thought that after my two Master's, I would surely get a job. But it was difficult. I applied for two jobs at the Institute, one was for the post of a Disability Officer and one was for a Cataloguer in the Institute's library, which I knew so well. I went to a de-brief session and was told that I had the qualification, but lacked experience! For the job of Cataloguing, one did not need speech! Nobody would give a job because of my speech. (The catch 22 is that without experience, I would never get a job. But again clearly the Institute was not ready for people like me.) I did not get the jobs.

I applied for many jobs. Some called me for interviews, some did not bother. I felt that my speech was the biggest barrier. The actual fact is that employers could see only my disability, not my capability. In any job, one requires speech and a limited amount of hand function. I did not get any job.

It was a terrible period in my life. I thought, 'Is this London, where I've grown-up, studied? I have two MAs'. I got de-motivated. It was the worst period in my life. I felt like a loser. Nikhil kept telling me to write and I decided to write. (I had a mind-set that I would never get a job due to the severity of my speech; it took me years to accept my limitations.) I had come a full circle. I was faced with this again. So, being the

Indian rubber ball I am, I bounced back. I put all my energy into writing.

'Dad, I want to do a course in Citylit', I said browsing the website.

'What is the point of doing so many writing courses', said dad as he accompanied me to enrol on yet another writing course.

'Writing courses help to bounce back ideas. You can't just sit and gape in front of the computer screen waiting for some brilliant brainwave to descend on you. Instead, I meet people and exchange ideas', I said with conviction.

'Okay', said dad. His okay was to really tell me to shut up as he went back to his favourite pastime of reading the *Economic Times*! 'We will go on Monday', he said.

I was encouraged, because in one of the first courses that I attended, Stacy, a fellow writer said to me, 'You are a writer first, and then you are disabled'. Just what I needed to hear. I never did let my handicap get me down for long. I would always know how to enjoy life.

On one occasion, I was feeling a bit bored with the hum-drum of life, so I joined a Scrabble Club (I managed to find one online) at the Royal Festival Hall at South Bank. I went and began playing. To my glee, I came third, beating a few of the Brits at it! I developed a new technique of using the mobile as a communicator and this worked. Rather than lugging my big communicator along everywhere behind my back, I used my mobile. This summer when I was in London, I went to an Indian shop round the corner from our home in Pimlico. They obviously did not understand my speech, so I texted what I wanted to buy—parathas, and the shopkeepers immediately understood me and got them for me. They took the change from my purse and put the parathas in a plastic bag and bid me a friendly goodbye.

'I was having one of my boring days in London. I was browsing through *Time Out*, and spotted a new theatre called Soho Theatre. It was showing an interesting play. With my speech impairment, and Vimla's lack of language skills, it doubly disabled me. I took my communicator and managed to get two tickets, for Bobbie and me. Bobbie and *mashi* were girl guides together at the United Nations. Bobbie had been a friend of our family ever since I was born. A disabled person gets concession tickets at half-price, and also for the attendant.

Once, I just felt like seeing a film—which film and where was unplanned. I jumped on to the usual 24 Bus which stops outside our flat in Pimlico. There was a bus divergence at Westminster so I had to get off. The whole of Trafalgar Square was being shut off. I slowly made my way to Leicester Square which was buzzing with life as usual. I went and wandered around. A Film called *You, Me and Dupree* was on. I went and asked how much was the fare. They understood my speech! It was £12. No way was I spending that amount of money. I mumbled that I will come back instead! I went to Trocadero only to find out that the chair lift was not working. I spied the Prince Charles Cinema hall close by and noticed that there was a film called *Lake House* that I wanted to see. It was my kind of film; I waited around until the doors opened. I went up to an usher and told him that I wanted to see the film and pointed to *Lake House*. The man called the film attendant, who quickly came. She was friendly. I bought my ticket and she told me to come back at 4.15 pm. I had half an hour to kill, so I went to a bar called, All Bar One and bought myself a Pims No. 1. The waitress took the change from my bag. Then I began looking for the loos. The waitress apologized that there were no loos with disability access in that bar. So, I went to the Mexican Restaurant Chiquotio. Two men had to come out with a folding ramp. I felt bad about that but I went in, performed and came back! Then finally, I went to The Prince Charles cinema hall, where I was taken in. The film was good. To return home I hailed a cab, and got in. Nearer home, I asked the cab driver to stop and I got out from the cab and paid the driver. He took the exact change from my purse. I asked him to help me put on my earphones of my ipod and off I wandered homeward bound. I walked home through the Embankment. It was my favourite walk home, passing through the Houses of Parliament Westminster Abbey, the Embankment Gardens, through Mill Bank Towers, through Tate Britain and Pimlico Gardens and then home. I felt very happy with myself.

Such magnificent architecture, bliss it was to be alive, but to be in London, was heavenly!

My cousin Suro was with us for a while. I met him at Trafalgar Square. First question he asked me was 'Where is Vimla?' He was really amazed that I had come there on my own. He had never seen me alone in his life!

It was in 2005 that I started lecturing at the Institute of Education. My mind went back to a day when I was finishing my dissertation at the Institute of Education. Gregg and I decided to have dinner out.

Gregg said in his usual loud fashion, 'Shall we call Felicity?' Felicity Armstrong is a prolific writer and academic on Inclusive Education. She was a renowned Professor. She had written hundreds of articles on disability and particularly, the social model of disability. I thought to myself, 'Would such a famous woman have dinner with us?'

I was envious at Gregg as he lectured on the course. I wanted to, but I thought my speech would be in the way yet again. I was getting a little disheartened. Everything needed speech and my speech sounded child-like and infantile.

As soon as she met me she said, 'I have read your dissertation and liked it immensely. I would love you to give a lecture, at the Institute to my students'. Wow! I could not believe this!

'I would be delighted to', I said. Though I was ecstatic I was going to lecture, I was but nervous because of my poor speech. I had learnt to create PowerPoint presentations at the London Met, so I did not have to speak much and any friend could read out the contents. Sometimes, I take a friend as an interpreter, so I took my friend Judy Larsen. Judy had done her PhD with mother but was especially friendly with me. She read out my power point presentations after which the students asked questions.

I have now developed a lecturing technique of putting up my entire lecture on a PowerPoint. Yes, obviously I felt self-conscious of my speech. I absolutely abhor the sound of my monotonous voice. I wish I had a sexy, husky one with a clipped Oxonian accent, but I guess one cannot have everything in life.

Students and academics are eager to know the inside perspective of a disabled person, from a disabled person. Anyway, believe it or not, I was a success. I began lecturing in India too. The current trend in the disability movement is for voices of disabled people to be heard. The next year, I was invited again. This carried on for five years. In the second or third year, there was a student from Paris who I had lectured to, Anne, who came up to me and said,

'Will you come and give a lecture at the Sorbonne University?' I could not believe this. No one in my family of academics had done this!

'Yes I would love to', I said giving her a big smile. I thought it would never materialize, but it did. Anne and I exchanged emails back and forth during that year. Before leaving for London for the summer I got my visa. My friend Theresa filled the visa form painstakingly. I went for the interview and got the visa.

'Hi, are you still interested in going to Paris?', I asked Susan as we walked towards a pub near the Milbank. I have been invited to lecture at the Sorbonne!

'Yes, of course, I am definitely coming', she said. She said she will not be missing this opportunity!

Dad bought the tickets for us. Mother came as well. We met Susan at Waterloo. She was on time for a change. I keep teasing her about her punctuality. When I was in IOE, I used to wait endlessly for her. However, she was on time, just about! We boarded the train, it had a portable ramp. I was travelling first—all disabled people are put in the first class with the attendant who was Susan. Mother smuggled her way into the first class. She said she would not need to eat or drink! The hostess smiled and said it was perfectly alright. 'You can get away with anything if you are charming.' We were all given a glass of Champagne each as we approached the Tour de Eiffel (including mother!).

Paris is a 'walking city'. One walks everywhere. This was the second time that Susan, mother and I were in Paris together.

Mother had taken us when I had finished my first dissertation. We had three whole days of fun, just strolling around and imbibing the beauty. Our favourite place was the Rodin Museum which had a beautiful café.

My Sorbonne lecture took place on a Tuesday. We met Anne at 11 o'clock and went through my presentation. I was to have two interpreters. Susan was going to translate what I said in English and Anne was going to translate in French. We had a gourmet lunch which Anne took us for and then we navigated our way to Sorbonne University.

It was an old dilapidated building, hundreds of years old. We spent about 20 minutes just finding an accessible entrance. Eventually, we found the lecture room. The Parisian students rolled in one by one. My presentation began. It took 20 minutes. After my presentation, the students all began to ask me questions. I then did the second 20 minutes. The lecture lasted for one-and-a-half hours! Questions kept coming. Some were personal; some were out of curiosity about the subject. None of the students had met a disabled adult. In the world today, there is a scarcity of us severely disabled people in the public domain. Previously, I used to get upset when people asked me how I coped with life as a disabled person, but as I got more empowered, I knew I will always be a rare specimen and so was always ready to respond to the questions. But the lecture confirmed that the world was beginning to accept us—they did not look at us as if we had come from Mars!

Over the years, Professor Armstrong or Felicity as she insisted on being called, and I became good friends.

'Happy birthday', said Felicity as she kissed me.

'Let's go for a drink to the Russell Hotel', she said.

On my 40th birthday she decided to take me to the Russell Hotel. This was going to be a special treat. The Russell Hotel was a very expensive one next to Russell Square. The Hotel had been the hub of the Bloomsbury Group, there was also a Virginia Woolf Café.

We trotted off only to be confronted by stairs at the entrance.

'Do you have a ramp?', asked Felicity politely.

'At the back of the building.'

'Why don't you have a ramp at the front of the Building?', said Felicity.

'No, well it's an old heritage building. We can't afford to ruin the décor', said the Porter. What an excuse!

'It's the law that every building in England should be accessible', said Felicity.

Nevertheless, we trudged to the back entrance and were taken up by the goods lift. My friend was seething with annoyance. She thought it was awful for disabled people to go up in a goods lift. We finally entered this grand building and walked to the bar which was really posh.

The Concierge came up and asked Felicity, 'How long are you going to stay?' I was so used to being questioned by the normal world that I thought it was a perfectly normal question, but for my academic friend this question was outrageous, invading privacy!

'How dare they ask us how long we were going to stay?'

'As long it takes to get drunk', answered Felicity, furious at their audacity at asking us how long we wanted to stay.

Despite the initial hiccup, we had two glasses of champagne, and ate some salmon, thoroughly enjoying each others company.

'Thank you. That was the best treat', I said, 'for my birthday'. 'Memorable'.

A wonderful 40th birthday with a wonderful friend, whose approach was always a level playing field!

I Get Employed!

Despite my two Master's, I had not got a job in London, not through want of trying but I felt sure, because of my disability. Most jobs need speech and my speech was not the world's best. It goes without saying that I would have preferred a BBC accent.

It was a warm September morning in 2006. I was ensconced in London, in my flat in Pimlico. I was half asleep, half awake. It was an unearthly hour in the morning when I heard a message on the voice mail. I could not believe what I heard. I replayed the answer phone to hear the melodious voice of my mother to make sure I was not hallucinating.

I rang her mobile. She was in Delhi on work, staying at the India International Centre where we usually stayed.

'Molls, I think you have a job. It's to be a Senior Event's Manager at the Oxford Bookstore in Mumbai', said mother excitedly.

What I had heard was correct.

'The owner of Oxford Bookstore was very impressed with your CV and said that you are fully qualified to be an Event Manager', mother explained. Mother went on to explain about the job. I wondered how I was going do the job with my poor speech. The more I heard, the more anxious I became.

I had to go to Delhi for the interview. On the day before the interview, my whole family was giving me mock interviews. I think they were more nervous than me. On the day itself, I had two interpreters. Yes, I was nervous as we drove along the chaotic Delhi roads to the office in Aurangzeb Road. Atiya and Varsha were with me. The interview lasted for about 45 minutes. Preeti Paul (they were the Pauls of the Apeejay Group) directed all the questions at me, which was a pleasant change. She seemed very liberal and enlightened. In fact, because she lived in London and India, like me, she was very open to giving me a chance.

I got the job (!)... in good old India. Unbelievable.

The next thing was how would I be able to do the job? I was supposed to increase the footfalls (revenue) in the bookshop through book launches and interesting talks. I had to organize four events a week. It took me some time to network with authors. This I did through chat, Facebook and email. Karuna put me onto Facebook, which revolutionized my life.

My one little finger again came up tops! I was very successful. I had eminent authors and well-known citizens of Bombay responding to my emails coming into Oxford to talk about their books. Theresa, my friend, helped me as my assistant, in making calls and negotiating with the authors. She had a lovely voice, spoke very well and helped to co-ordinate whatever I directed and planned. It is vital for a disabled person to have an assistant. With an assistant, disabled people can perform the job to their fullest potential. In England and US, disabled people have this service when employed. I know someone who had four (!) in the US. I received a great deal of support also from my friends, Sumita Sen and Varsha Hooja during the events. I would develop an event, co-ordinate it, get it started and Sumita and Varsha would be happy to introduce the authors and thank them on my behalf. Everyone accepted this as a norm. They realized that this was happening due to my poor speech. I interacted with my colleagues through G Chat. During my early days, there was a quick turnover of managers; I had a tough time convincing every new manager that I could think. It took months each time, after which it was time for the next change.

I think what made a difference is that because I had grown up here in Bombay, people knew me. Obviously I was popular, they liked me. Their response to the events I planned was very heartening. Through successful events, the elite and the intelligentsia saw that I had a brain. I bounced back to life. I had written a lot and of course I was not invisible.

I was employable. After my return, I was also able to bring in attitudinal changes through the group, which I had earlier formed called ADAPT (an acronym for Able Disabled All People Together). The matter of rights of disabled people had taken a centre stage all over the world. Disabled people today in the West were in the forefront of all decision-making and were involved in the running of disability organizations. 'Nothing about us, without us' was the current thinking all over the world.

I had become the trustee of the organization which had 15 members on the Governing Body scrutinizing the Society's functioning within the Charity Commissioner's Laws. I decided to review the objectives of ADAPT. I had initially started it as a recreational club for people with disabilities and able-bodied people, designed on the basis of the PHAB Clubs in

Britain. When I left for England in 1993, the social meetings slowly dwindled down to no meeting. No one felt the need to activate it until 2000, when I returned to India again.

In India, the Persons with Disabilities (PWD) Act was passed in 1995. Both *mashi* and dad were instrumental and were a part of the formation committee. The aim and objective of ADAPT was to ensure accessibility, equal opportunity, equal participation as defined in the PWD.

After mother's PhD, the Spastics Society of India had embarked on a Project with Canada. The Indo-Canadian project dealt primarily with mainstreaming disabled adults and children into society to make it more inclusive. As part of the Canadian project, the Society needed to form a disability activist group focusing on rights and entitlements, in keeping with the global trend, 'Nothing about us, without us'.

'What should be the topic of conference?' asked mother when we were discussing a conference to be held.

'Why not have it on the theme of citizenship?', said Nilesh who had been to school to the Centre for Special Education with me and had read my essay on 'Citizenship and Barriers'.

'Yes, a very good idea', said the group. Neenu and Sunita, women with disabilities, had joined our new group. The conference was a huge success. Micheal Bach and Vianne Timmons, our Canadian partners, along with Diana Leonard, flew down for the conference as did my uncle (*mesho*) from Delhi. The outcome of the conference was the formation of ADAPT's Rights Group (ARG). This Rights Group differed from other disability groups in that ADAPT included both non-disabled and disabled people. We believed that both 'able' and 'disabled' should work together to form an 'inclusive' society where 'all' are welcome and included. We activists strongly condemned the segregation of disabled persons in 'ghettoized' organizations, made up of only disabled people. We (the ARG team) believed that this attitude is yet another expression of exclusion that further hinders the creation of a truly inclusive society. The three main objectives of ADAPT were to initiate change in access, attitude and policy for people with disabilities in India. The central message of ARG has been 'Nothing about us, without us'. ARG recognized that without a wide collective recognition of people with disability and an acknowledgement of their human rights, there will be no public and political will or lobby for change. It was unanimously agreed that I become the Chairperson of ADAPT, with Anita Prabhu, as co-Chairperson. Nilesh, Neenu and Sunita became founder members. Amena was appointed to build a database of the alumni.

The most critical phrase of feminist theory and practice is, perhaps, the statement that 'personal is political', that what happens in private, is power-based and it should not be secret or concealed. It should be spoken about in public in a political manner and that collective action can be taken to change it. So I used my personal experiences of inaccessibility into the public forefront, getting more ramps and making Bombay more accessible.

The achievements were made in various ways. We filed many Public Interest Litigations (PILs) against the state of Maharashtra for non-implementation of the PWD Act. We conducted Access Audits of public places, appealing to the authorities to make inaccessible places disabled friendly. As a result of ARG's lobbying, hospitals, multiplex cinema halls, shopping malls and amusement parks became disabled friendly. A personal touch of actually meeting the people concerned and talking to us helped. But there were terrible times too. Once I had gone shopping for Diwali with Pam. The shop-keeper banned my wheelchair in one of the sections of the shop saying that the shop was too narrow and wheelchairs were not allowed. Everyone stared at us at the entrance. It was a leading store in Breach Candy, Bombay. We left feeling very humiliated. But not for long. When we reached The Spastics Society of India, they were outraged and in the next few days, we gathered together at least 50 people on wheelchairs and had a demonstration outside the shop. The traffic police supporting us, diverted the traffic and the road outside the shop was pedestrianized. The shop did not know what hit them. Our demonstration was a huge success. The owner of the shop initially refused to come out, but with our shouting he came out and apologized and said we were his children (!) and invited us, in-all 50 of us on wheelchairs. It caused immense publicity. We also got many calls from friends who had read about it in the press saying that it was the best thing we had done.

Another example of our might was in 2005, a memorable year for us.

In 2004, we were denied entry to the Mumbai Marathon. The rules stated 'No wheelchair vehicles or dogs allowed on the course'. Unimaginable but true. We began a huge agitation. My brother played a crucial role—he joined us and began fighting the authorities. We approached our patron, Mr Sunil Dutt, who was then the Sports Minister at the Centre and he was so upset about our exclusion that he promptly rang up the State Sports Minister. The Marathon organizers were asked to stop the event or include wheelchair users. On 16 January 2005, a landmark event allowed wheelchair participants to run the Standard

Chartered Mumbai Marathon for the first time in India. Placards with 'You see disability, I see ability; You see a wheelchair, I see investment' were all over the place.

We have become quite well-known now and quite feared as well with our demonstrations, lobbies, articles in the media, et cetera. I did not know I could be an activist. More recently, I have been focusing on empowering disabled people and sensitizing corporates to hire employees with disability. I wrote articles and brochures on 'Does inclusion matter? How inclusive are we?' I targeted the electronic and print media. I began writing articles. Few of them are—'Are You Alone'; 'Where Is Your Helper?'; 'Citizenship and the Links Between the Different Models of Disability'; 'Does She Take Sugar In Her Tea?'; 'From Charity to Rights: A Cross Cultural Perspective'; 'I may be different but aren't we all?'; 'Society creates a Norm and the norm excludes disabled people'; 'Voices of people in special schools', et cetera.

For the organization (ADAPT), I used my internet skills, which had been honed in the course at the London Met and created a global internet Chat Forum. The forum provided a platform for sharing information and resources. This brought up issues of loneliness, marriage, sex and growing old without parents.

What is most exciting about my job is that I can do it from wherever I am, as a lot of it is done online. This is my strength. It is also exciting because my work gives me the space to continue my other passion: giving talks at the Institute of Education and conducting courses there from time to time.

I began designing a special Empowerment Course which is my interpretation of the new social model, where I combined my studies of Feminist and Disability Theories. I put in Law and Disability. The Empowerment Courses are for people with disability with the aim of enabling everyone to understand good practices of inclusion and the PWD Act. I began lecturing in the Training and Pedagogy Department of ADAPT to students of the Teacher Training Course and students of the Community Initiatives in Inclusive Education (CIIE) coming from different parts of the world like Mongolia, Tonga, Chile, Bangladesh, Pakistan and of course, India. I began conducting Empowerment Courses in Bombay, Delhi and am doing one this year in Jharkhand and Gujarat. When I began lecturing in Bombay, students wanted me to present my lecture on a PowerPoint on my own—they said they did not require an interpreter.

I am now thoroughly busy. I have the job at Oxford and my work with ARG. I am involved in my Empowerment Courses.

Reflections

I have used the one little finger 50,000 times! This strenuous, exhausting and exhilarating journey is coming to a close. My first book is almost over. Unbelievable! It has been an emotional upheaval revisiting my life. Now as I pen my last chapter, I am introspective.

With a disheartening beginning as a child who got singled out, life has not always been a cakewalk. Yet I have surmounted many obstacles. The doctor who said I would be a permanent vegetable has had to eat his words. I have two Master's degrees. I travel, write and lecture across India and abroad. I was asked to leave shops and canteens because I was in a wheelchair, but today I go shopping on my own in London, and regularly eat out with friends at restaurants in Bombay, Delhi, Paris and London. They said '*I think these people should be locked up*'. Today we are visible everywhere—in movie theatres, restaurants, schools, universities, parks—you name it. Make it accessible and you will see us there! Existing laws have ruled in our favour. While some nations honour and implement these laws and some do not, I stand witness to change—to insurmountable obstacles becoming challenges that can be conquered. We are not at the top of the mountain yet, there is much more to be done but we are on the road—and now there is no stopping our journey.

I am thankful that my life and my body have made me philosophical. I think the art of living, lies not just in confronting our troubles but minimizing them and focusing on the positive aspects of our life. Most of us are swimming against the tide of trouble in, what I think of as, the ocean of our life. Yet we need to survive, make it to the shore and not let the waves engulf us. I feel I have managed to do that, with the steady support of my family who fought the battle along with me. The struggle to overcome adversity has made me a tough survivor in a family of brave soldiers.

As I reflect back, I realize that the move to England was essential for mother and me to survive and was a wise move on the part of my parents. It was also equally essential for us to return to India. Perhaps it was destined, as this return started the disability movement in India and helped other disabled children gain access to education. I do feel euphoric that my need for a special school has benefited other disabled children in India.

I write this last chapter as I sit in Russell Square gazing at the undulating grass, flowers in full bloom, toddlers hopping in and out of the water fountain under the watchful eye of their mothers. I watch a boy playing in the fountain and wonder what life has in store for him. Behind me is Russell Hotel. It still seems inviting, with architecture that will always remain magnificent. The square looks ravishing! I think to myself—how I love nature and the peaceful beauty of London Parks and this beloved square. How fortunate I am that my life has been an east-west journey, a privilege that not many have. My early link with the West was critical and it greatly benefited my growth and personality. It was in England that my parents found out

I could think! In later years, it was the available communication technology and strategies in this nurturing environment, which empowered and helped me to overcome my communication difficulties and also encouraged me to question. Learning about the latest social model of disability and the changing approach to the treatment of disabled people helped me to accept my own challenging situation and my body. Later in India, it helped mother and me to take the fledgling disability movement forward. There is no doubt that my early and ongoing exposure to the West has had a major impact on my growth and empowerment.

Today, my articles are published in the local papers. They educate the public—making them aware that disabled people are not children. Disabled adults have adult thoughts, desires, feelings, passions, views and expectations like other 'normal' adults. But most of the time these desires remain unquenched. People are not willing to look past our bodies into our souls. People (especially in India) see us as children and children should not be heard. They look at our imperfect bodies, and believe some of the religious beliefs which explain that we are the way we are, due to a retribution for past sins committed. I wonder seriously sometimes—what is the sin I committed?

I must admit that in London, I am free of all this negative thinking. I do not feel so disabled there. I am independent. I go to the supermarket for the daily shopping, stop at the launderette, the chemist, buy the best fish for mother (a Bengali addicted to her *maach* or fish) from the local farmers market. Doing all this makes me so pleased with myself. That joy of freely moving around on my own, emotionally feeling needed and of contributing is immediately snatched away from me as

I hit Bombay's dusty airport. There will be no more moving around on my own. The roads are full of potholes, there are hardly any pavements; most shops, libraries, theatres, cinema halls, restaurants, bookshops and museums are inaccessible. I know I will be paralyzed at home.

There will of course be those whispers and piercing stares (Indians seem to have made staring a national habit). Those endless painful questions, the rejections. The little oppressions of not being able to converse with me or treating me as an outcaste or an invisible individual will continue. I will still be looked upon as a child because of my speech and body. I want to scream and tell them that I am a 42 year old woman!

Attitudes *do matter*. They can make you feel included or excluded. Even today, many who do not know me, or have never met a disabled person in their life will automatically address the person I am with. They will talk about me in front of me but never with me! They will follow this up with '*can she hear*' '*Does she understand*' or '*She went to Oxford? How nice!*' The conversation then comes to a screeching halt. They have nothing more to say. Even today, many will invite the whole family for dinner or a party but not me! Do they feel I am infectious? Are they ashamed? I yearn for my friends, my social network. I yearn for the people who accept me. I long to breathe. I long for the openness of life.

Why do I feel so small, so isolated so rejected in India? Why do I yearn after a few months to run back to where they treat me as a human being? *Will I make it?* is a question that nags me. I get into a panic. Life means freedom. Freedom to think, move, speak, interact with whomsoever, freedom to make choices. Without this, it is not life. One does not live. One only exists. Getting back means the loss of it. Initially there would be those tears. Gradually I would begin to analyze, I would reason with my mind.

Today, my mind takes over. I do not want to be normal! I feel just like everyone else, yet that does not seem to be the case in the eyes of this society. Previously, I would have liked to have got married. That was a period of 'normalization'. I had to be normal. Foucault argues *who is normal?'* and, *'who is disabled?' 'Who decides normal and abnormal?'*. Are we conditioned by society in the definition of what is normal? Do we only see it from society's perspective of normalization? Or can the definitions evolve as time goes by to include everyone? Is everyone perfect? I may never have a man to hold me or a child of my own and never be in a traditional situation. I realize I will always continue to struggle. Adjust to the reality of people shunning me will be a lifelong challenge. To minimize and to accept life as it is, is a discipline like yoga which I regularly do. I have grown and developed in an atmosphere where there has been control of thinking, of my own self, of the mind over the body, of the spirit over the physical, just so adequately put by Emerson,

What lies behind us and what lies before us are tiny matters compared to what lies within us. (Ralph Waldo Emerson)

And those tears dry up. Having experienced acceptance and rejection, I turn to the positive aspects of my life. I tell myself how fortunate I am because not many can live the way I have and the way I do. I am fortunate to have friends who reach out to me and love me. I cherish those friends who love me just the way I am. They do not try and make your kind of 'normal' which I can never be or may not want to be, because I do not know what your 'normal' is. I know only *me*. I like me.

I have learned to love and accept that *life is beautiful* as it is. It is not always easy, but definitely beautiful. I think that despite the attitudes of rejection, lack of access and the loss of freedom, I have accepted India as home. No matter how hard it may be to live in India, it will always be home, and I will always return home. I am comfortable now in the light and the dark, the smiles and the tears.

Yet a part of me will always belong to London. The opportunity to be a part of life in London is the nectar in my jar, the honey in the flower and the rainbow in the storm. As long as I have a taste of that nectar on a regular basis, I have found strength to salute life and live it with laughter and humour.

I am like the migrating bird with her freedom to spend the winter months away and the summer at home. The hybrid, nurtured and fed by two cultures, aware of both the joy of being accepted and the pain of rejection. Trying to remember to live life one day at a time and to accept who I am. Hoping to rise upto the struggle and challenge of doing so against a sea of apathy and rejection. Living, hoping and believing that there is a better tomorrow. Finally free to be *me*.